Recent Results in Cancer Research 103

Recent Results in Cancer Research

Volume 95: Spheroids in Cancer Research
Edited by H. Acker, J. Carlsson, R. Durand, R. M. Sutherland
1984. 83 figures, 12 tables. IX, 183. ISBN 3-540-13691-6

Volume 96: Adjuvant Chemotherapy of Breast Cancer
Edited by H.-J. Senn
1984. 98 figures, 91 tables. X, 243. ISBN 3-540-13738-6

Volume 97: Small Cell Lung Cancer
Edited by S. Seeber
1985. 44 figures, 47 tables. VII, 166. ISBN 3-540-13798-X

Volume 98: Perioperative Chemotherapy
Edited by U. Metzger, F. Largiadèr, H.-J. Senn
1985. 48 figures, 45 tables. XII, 157. ISBN 3-540-15124-9

Volume 99: Peptide Hormones in Lung Cancer
Edited by K. Havemann, G. Sorenson, C. Gropp
1985. 100 figures, 63 tables. XII, 248. ISBN 3-540-15504-X

Volume 100:
Therapeutic Strategies in Primary and Metastatic Liver Cancer
Edited by Ch. Herfarth, P. Schlag, P. Hohenberger
1986. 163 figures, 104 tables. ISBN 3-540-16011-6

Volume 101:
Locoregional High-Frequency Hyperthermia and Temperature Measurement
Edited by G. Bruggmoser, W. Hinkelbein, R. Engelhardt, M. Wannenmacher
1986. 96 figures, 8 tables. IX, 143. ISBN 3-540-15501-5

Volume 102: Epidemiology of Malignant Melanoma
Edited by R. P. Gallagher
1986. 15 figures, 70 tables, IX, 169. ISBN 3-540-16020-5

Preoperative (Neoadjuvant) Chemotherapy

Edited by
J. Ragaz, P. R. Band, and J. H. Goldie

With 58 Figures and 49 Tables

Springer-Verlag
Berlin Heidelberg New York Tokyo

Joseph Ragaz, M. D.
Pierre R. Band, M. D.
James H. Goldie, M. D.

Cancer Control Agency of British Columbia
600 West 10th Avenue
Vancouver, B. C. V5Z 4E6, Canada

ISBN-13: 978-3-642-82673-3 e-ISBN-13: 978-3-642-82671-9
DOI: 10.1007/978-3-642-82671-9

Library of Congress Cataloging-in-Publication Data. Main entry under title: Preoperative (neoadjuvant) chemotherapy. (Recent results in cancer research; 103) Includes bibliographies and index. 1. Cancer-Adjuvant treatment. 2. Preoperative care. I. Ragaz, J. (Joseph), 1945- . II. Band, P. R. (Pierre R.), 1935- . III. Goldie, James H. IV. Series. [DNLM: 1. Adjuvants, Immunologic-therapeutic use. 2. Adjuvants, Pharmaceutic-therapeutic use. 3. Neoplasms-drug therapy. 4. Preoperative Care.
W1 RE106P v. 103/QZ 267 P927] RC261.R35 vol. 103 616.99'4 s
[616.99'4061] 85-30312 [RC271.A35]

Softcover reprint of the hardcover 1st edition 1986

Typesetting, printing, and binding: Appl, Wemding
2125/3140-543210

Preface

Despite recent advances in adjuvant therapies of cancer, the regimens of postoperative adjuvant chemotherapy treatment which are presently available fail to cure the majority of cancer patients. Preoperative (neoadjuvant) chemotherapy represents a new approach in drug scheduling, based on sound theoretical, pharmacokinetic, and experimental principles.

The preoperative timing of chemotherapy before definitive surgery is not a minor change in the therapy of cancer. To be successful, large numbers of practitioners and their patients must participate. Substantial alterations of many aspects of the present management of cancer will have to follow. Therefore, before such therapy can be fully and routinely implemented, results of the novel treatment and its rationale have to be carefully evaluated.

In preoperative treatment, other features will likely gain importance. For the first time, clinicians have a chance to follow the in vivo response of the tumor exposed to preoperative chemotherapy. The subsequent histological assessment of the tumor sample may likely become an important prognostic guide, permitting more refined individual approaches to the planning of postoperative adjuvant treatment. The value of such a treatment strategy can already be appreciated in the clinical setting, as seen from the therapy of osteosarcoma. Furthermore, preoperative chemotherapy might render previously inoperable tumors operable and hence resectable with a curative intention. The preoperative reduction of tumor bulk may also effectively decrease the need for more radical operations, permitting a more uniform adoption of conservative surgery. Although the most important departure from conventional adjuvant treatment, the preoperative timing of chemotherapy is, therefore, not the only element of the neoadjuvant approach.

Our Vancouver symposium took place in March 1985. In organizing the convention we were greatly helped by a generous grant of Lederle Canada and their international branch, as well as by the competent assistance of Betty Fata and Lisa Lockerby from the conference organizing company Venue West. Invited speakers summarized the current preclinical and clinical aspects of neoadjuvant chemotherapy. The material presented represents an update and a comprehensive review of the key issues of the neoadjuvant therapy of cancer.

We hope that the present efforts and research on preoperative chemotherapy, as reflected in this volume, represent only a beginning rather than the end of what looks like a very promising approach towards the therapy of cancer.

Vancouver, Canada
December 1985

J. Ragaz
P. R. Band
J. H. Goldie

Contents

*List of Contributors**

* The adress of the principal author is given on the first page of each contribution

[1] Page on which contribution begins

Clinical and Scientific Considerations in Preoperative (Neoadjuvant) Chemotherapy

E. Frei III, D. Miller, J. R. Clark, B. G. Fallon, and T. J. Ervin

Dana-Farber Cancer Institute, 44 Binney Street, Boston, MA 02115, USA

Introduction

Thirty years ago, chemotherapy had little to offer patients with solid tumors and in general patients were treated after failure of surgery or radiotherapy when advanced overt metastatic disease was already present. As progress was made in the chemotherapy of the childhood solid tumors, and of certain adult tumors, such as metastatic breast cancer, the investigation of chemotherapy in the *adjuvant* situation developed. This was stimulated by the fact that, for example, patients with stage II breast cancer or osteogenic sarcoma are at high risk of having micrometastatic dissemination at the time of diagnosis, so that potentially definitive treatment must include not only control of the primary with surgery and/or radiotherapy (S/R), but also systemic chemotherapy (C), the latter to control disseminated micrometastatic disease. The experimental basis for this was the observation that chemotherapy for in vivo transplanted tumors was capable of cytoeradication (cure) in inverse relationship to the tumor burden. Thus chemotherapy which produced only partial regression of advanced tumor was frequently curative when applied to the same tumor in microscopic form (Goldin et al. 1956). This was also demonstrated in experimental in vivo systems, wherein the primary in the extremity was controlled by amputation, following which the cure rate could be increased in many circumstances by chemotherapy addressed to micrometastatic disease (Skipper 1978).

A more recent evolution of multidisciplinary treatment strategy has been the use of C initially, followed by S/R, in patients with solid tumors. The purpose of this approach is (1) to improve control of the primary by stage reduction and/or (2) to improve control of micrometastatic disease. Examples include head and neck cancer, where the major problem is control of the primary; breast cancer and osteogenic sarcoma, where the major problem is control of micrometastatic disease; and lung cancer, where control of both locoregional and disseminated micrometastatic disease is a major problem.

I have chosen the term "neoadjuvant chemotherapy" for this strategy (Frei 1982). It perpetuates the term "adjuvant" which, though it was an unfortunate choice, is thoroughly entrenched. Also, it is a hybrid of generic terms. I prefer "neoadjuvant," however, because it is unambiguous, in contrast to other terms, such as "preoperative chemotherapy," which leaves out the important discipline of radiotherapy, and "induction chemotherapy," which has an old and well-defined meaning, in the context of the leukemias. Neoadjuvant chemotherapy (NA-C) is not a novel strategy in a sense, since it was employed successfully 15-20 years ago in the multidisciplinary treatment of childhood solid tumors, and studies have been performed in the past of some adult solid tumors. However, it is new as a strategy for adult solid tumors, in the sense that progress in chemotherapy has made it an idea whose time has come.

Recent Results in Cancer Research. Vol 103

The importance and potential of neoadjuvant chemotherapy can be appreciated by the fact that failure of curative treatment for cancer (for the 50% not cured) is due to failure of control of the primary tumor in 40%, of micrometastatic disease in 60%, and of macrometastatic disease present at the time of diagnosis in 50%. These figures add up to more than 100%, since patients may fall into several categories.

Control of the Primary Tumor: Advantages for Neoadjuvant Chemotherapy

The major goal is maximally to shrink an advanced primary tumor, such that it becomes operable and/or subject to definitive treatment by radiotherapy (stage reduction). With improved neoadjuvant chemotherapy, it may become useful in treating patients with more limited primary tumors in terms of size, with the intent of decreasing the extent of surgery and/or radiotherapy which for some sites (head and neck cancer and extremity sarcomas) may provide major cosmetic and functional advantages.

Reduction of the primary tumor by chemotherapy, followed by surgery, provides a major opportunity for the study of the biology of solid tumors, particularly as perturbed by size reduction and/or by chemotherapy. The tumor can be compared with the initial biopsy and the nature of chemotherapy-induced tumor shrinkage in terms of pathology, stem cell biology, stromal-tumor cell relationships, and vascularity. In addition, the effects of chemotherapy on the tumor's persistence and qualitative characteristics at a morphologic, immunologic, differentiation, cytokinetic, and other levels could be studied. Of major practical importance is the issue as to whether tumor regression, as perceived by clinical and radiographic observation, results from an actual retraction of the tumor in terms of size, as compared with a decrease in tumor cell density and softening, which would represent cytoreduction but not a physical decrease in size of tumor. Preliminary observations suggest that either extreme of the above may occur with gradations in between. Clearly this has major implications for treatment strategy with S/R following C. It should be recalled that much of the progress in the treatment of leukemia 20-30 years ago was made possible by post-treatment examination of the bone marrow, wherein the effects of chemotherapy at a quantitative and qualitative level could be studied.

Another advantage for neoadjuvant chemotherapy is that chemotherapy is maximally effective when used early in the course of a given neoplastic disease. For example, Adriamycin produces a 50% response rate in patients with early metastatic breast carcinoma, but only a 15%-20% response rate in patients who have received prior chemotherapy. There is abundant evidence that prior surgery and particularly radiotherapy, which may compromise the vascularity and increase the heterogeneity of tumors, will adversely affect response to chemotherapy. Thus the use of chemotherapy initially provides the optimal circumstance for achieving response in overt neoplastic disease (Henderson et al. 1982).

Neoadjuvant chemotherapy provides an in vivo assay system for chemotherapy. Experimental studies indicate a high correlation between responsiveness of macrometastatic disease and micrometastatic disease for a given chemotherapy. Thus response of the primary tumor to chemotherapy may be expected to predict for responsiveness of micrometastatic disease and thus is of tactical importance for treating the individual patient. This area was pioneered for the neoadjuvant chemotherapy of osteogenic sarcoma (Rosen et al. 1984).

In addition to stage reduction, neoadjuvant chemotherapy provides additional favorable effects, particularly for radiotherapy. Thus, tumor size reduction would be associated with an increase in vascularity and therefore oxygen supply, which would increase the effectiveness of radiotherapy. Because of improved oxygenation and nutrient supply generally, as well as decrease in tumor cell density, the growth fraction of the regressed primary tumor should increase. Finally, some of the compounds employed in neoadjuvant chemotherapy, such as cisplatin, may have intrinsic radiosensitization properties.

There are certain potential and acutal disadvantages to the use of neoadjuvant chemotherapy. The primary and historical one was lack of effectiveness in terms of producing tumor regression. This problem has been solved for some tumors by improved chemotherapy. For example, tumor regression can be achieved in the majority of patients with head and neck cancer, stage III breast cancer, osteogenic sarcoma, and selected other tumors.

A second problem relates to the potential of selecting drug-resistant cells in the primary tumor, even while in the process of undergoing tumor regression. Experimental studies indicate that primary transplantable tumors, after they reach a given size, will regularly disseminate. Such dissemination is promptly controlled by chemotherapy, which causes regression of the primary, and even by chemotherapy which does not cause tumor regression but prevents further enlargement.

A final disadvantage of neoadjuvant chemotherapy with respect to the primary tumor relates to toxicity. Chemotherapy may affect the oral cavity, and thus potentially increase the toxicity of radiotherapy in head and neck cancer. Chemotherapy over a 2-month period may compromise nutrition. With proper supportive care, timing, and alimentation techniques, most of these problems can be effectively dealt with.

Control of Micrometastatic Disease by Neoadjuvant Chemotherapy

Primary treatment with surgery, and particularly with radiotherapy, with or without surgery, may incur a 1- to 4-month delay befor systemic treatment with chemotherapy is initiated. There is experimental evidence that such a delay may be critical, particularly in terms of drug resistance. Elsewhere in this volume, Drs. Goldie, Coldman, and Skipper will discuss drug resistance. By mathematical modeling and as confirmed in biological systems, it has been found that within five doublings, or less than a 2-log increase in the microscopic burden, the risk of drug-resistant mutant cells may increase from 5% to 95%. In experimental transplanted tumors, the doubling time of microscopic or small tumors may be a matter of a few days, after which, as the tumor increases in size, the doubling time is progressively lengthened because of cell loss and decreased growth fraction (Gompertzian curve). There is evidence, particularly by cytokinetic extrapolation, that the doubling time of microscopic human tumors may be shorter than that of their overt counterpart (Shackney et al. 1978). Having said this, it should be emphasized that we know preciously little about the biology of human micrometastases. Certainly by extrapolation, clonal evolution due to mutations, with progressive heterogeneity, may be assumed. While the potential for stem cell self-renewal would be expected to be high in microscopic tumors, that is, approaching 1, which would make them highly sensitive to chemotherapy, it is also possible that the opposite is true. Dvorak has demonstrated that microscopic metastases may exist in fibrin "cocoons," protected from the host for relatively long periods. Microscopic tumors may be indolent for substantial periods before tumor angiogenesis factor is produced and exponential growth occurs. There is recent evidence from Alexander that certain experimental microscopic metastases may have long periods of indolence (very low growth fraction). Finally, late metastases, particularly in breast cancer, but other solid tumors as well, are hard to reconcile with early cytokinetically aggressive microscopic metastases. However, it is not essential that indolent tumors in terms of time to relapse be cytokinetically quiescent. For example, if the potential for self-renewal of stem cells approaches 1, the tumor will grow rapidly and exponentially. To the extent that the stem cell self-renewal capacity approaches 50%, which is probably true for many tumors, growth would be substantially delayed. In summary, studies of the natural history of human micrometastatic disease are very much needed, and the biology of such tumors may be revealed by well-constructed clinical trials. Certainly, at face value, the phenomenon of clonal evolution in in vitro experimental systems and certain clinical trials, such as those of Nissen-Meyer, strongly support therapeutic trials that involve the earliest possible treatment of micrometastatic disease.

Clinical Examples of Neoadjuvant Chemotherapy

Although studies of neoadjuvant chemotherapy for head and neck cancer require confirmation and extension, there is increasing evidence that such treatment may improve long-term disease-free survival for advanced stage III and IV patients with head and neck cancer. Head and neck cancer, which represents a common epithelial tumor, has proven highly responsive initially to chemotherapy. Thus combinations involving cisplatin and fluorouracil (FU) or cisplatin plus bleomycin plus methotrexate have produced tumor regression in 70%-90% of patients and complete clinical and radiographic response in some 30%-50% of patients (Ervin et al. 1981). Thus this tumor is highly responsive, at least initially, to chemotherapy. This of itself has major importance. Secondly, it has been found that the presence and magnitude of response to neoadjuvant chemotherapy markedly affects disease-free survival following surgery and/or radiotherapy. Indeed, by multistep regression analysis of all prognostic factors, it has been found, after appropriate adjustment, that patients who achieve complete response with neoadjuvant chemotherapy have an improved disease-free survival as compared with patients who do not respond or have a partial response ($P = 0.0004$). Thus the production of a good response, that is, stage reduction by neoadjuvant chemotherapy, has a powerful and independent effect on prognosis. Further strategies are: (1) a comparative study of neoadjuvant chemotherapy versus a standard control and (2) improved neoadjuvant chemotherapy with the intent to increase the complete response rate, since this correlates with survival. Improving the complete response rate should result from increasing the number of neoadjuvant courses of chemotherapy from two to a maximum of four, since many patients are in the dynamic process of responding after one to two courses. Further combinations of chemotherapy, particularly those involving concurrent platinum and FU with interposed methotrexate with leucovorin rescue may prove more effective. Biological studies of the surgically resected specimen after chemotherapy should determine the risk of local recurrence, and hence the likelihood that postoperative (standard) chemotherapy will be needed. Finally, studies of tumor biology, drug effects, and drug resistance as indicated above, both for the primary and for micrometastatic disease, should have a major impact on future approaches to the neoadjuvant chemotherapy of head and neck cancer.

Finally, subsequently in this volume, important studies of neoadjuvant chemotherapy relating to a variety of diseases, such as stages II and III breast cancer; mesenchymal tumors, such as osteogenic sarcoma and soft tissue sarcoma; squamous cell carcinomas, not unlike head and neck, such as esophageal, cervical, and anal carcinoma; an finally regional stage III lung, are highly important, since for almost all of these diseases, progress in chemotherapy has occurred, and there is variable evidence that the neoadjuvant approach may provide a major increment in therapy. Lessons learned from these diseases, as well as from head and neck cancer, and particularly from basic tumor biology and pharmacology, will be interrelated and complementary. Neoadjuvant chemotherapy is here to stay and is a strategy which will provide major increments in cancer therapy, particularly against some of the more common forms of cancer, in the immediate future.

References

Ervin RJ, Weichselbaum RR, Miller D, Meshad M, Posner MR, Fabian RL (1981) Treatment of advanced squamous cell carcinoma of the head and neck with cisplatin, bleomycin and methotrexate (PBM). Cancer Treat Rep 65: 797-791

Frei E III (1982) Clinical cancer research: an embattled species. Cancer 50: 1979-1992

Goldin A, Venditti J, Humphreys S, Mantel N (1956) Influence of concentration of leukemic inoculum on the effectiveness of treatment. Science 123: 840

Henderson IC, Gelman R, Parker LM, et al (1982) 15 vs. 30 weeks of adjuvant chemotherapy for breast cancer patients with a high risk of recurrence: a randomized trial. Proc Am Soc Clin Oncol 1: 75

Rosen G, Marcove RC, Huvos AG, et al (1984) Primary osteogenic sarcoma: 8-year experience with adjuvant chemotherapy. J Cancer Res Clin Oncol 106: 77-68

Shackney SE, McCormack GW, Cuchural GJ (1978) Growth rate patterns of solid tumors and their relationship to responsiveness to therapy. Ann Intern Med 89: 107-121

Skipper HE (1978) Adjuvant chemotherapy. Cancer 41: 936

Experimental Adjuvant Chemotherapy: An Overview

H. E. Skipper

Southern Research Institute, 2000 Ninth Avenue, South, Birmingham, AL 35255, USA

Introduction

By way of introduction, I will indicate in some detail what the *key words* in my assigned title mean to me.

Experimental Chemotherapy

All sorts of research in which single drugs or combinations of drugs are delivered in different ways - alone, or in conjunction with surgery or radiotherapy - to animals bearing various neoplasms at different stages of advancement and degrees of dissemination.

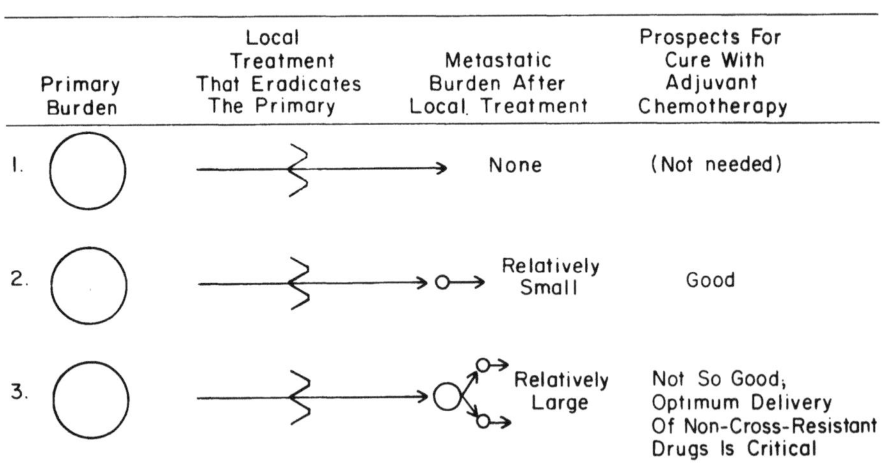

Fig. 1. The role of conventional adjuvant chemotherapy. The absence or presence of widely metastatic disease dictates curability by surgery or radiotherapy alone. The metastatic burden and the proportions of limiting T/R cells therein have a major influence on curability with adjuvant chemotherapy, as does the manner in which non-cross-resistant drugs are delivered. In experimental cancers where metastasis to "vital sites" is rapid and uniform in rate (after implantation), delay in local surgery for 1 week or more may result in no cures and little or no increase in survival time of surgical failures over untreated controls. In other experimental cancers where metastasis to vital sites is less rapid and less uniform, the situation is quite different

Recent Results in Cancer Research. Vol 103

For such research to be of major interest to me, the experiments must be conceived and designed in a manner that offers promise of gaining basic or pragmatic information that is relevant to problems faced in treating one or many human cancers. Quantitative information always has seemed especially important because treatment that reduces the tumor stem cell burden by, say, 99.9999%, although impressive, must be classified as failure. One or a few surviving tumor cells at the end of treatment may be too many.

The experimental systems we have used often are transplantable neoplasms in inbred mice: leukemias and lymphomas; osteogenic, lung, breast, colon, ovarian, and pancreatic tumors; malignant melanomas - and a few others. Using criteria similar to those employed at the clinical level, these experimental neoplasms may be classified as responsive, refractory, or very refractory to chemotherapy used alone or in an adjuvant setting.

One would have to be naive not to recognize the *quantitative differences* between experimental cancers, between human cancers, and between experimental and human cancers often make direct carryover of therapeutic protocols *impossible* without taking into consideration differences in tumor burden, growth rate, and, most important, stem cell heterogeneity, which affects the shapes and slopes of dose-response and time-action-response curves. On the other hand, few who have monitored both experimental and clinical re-

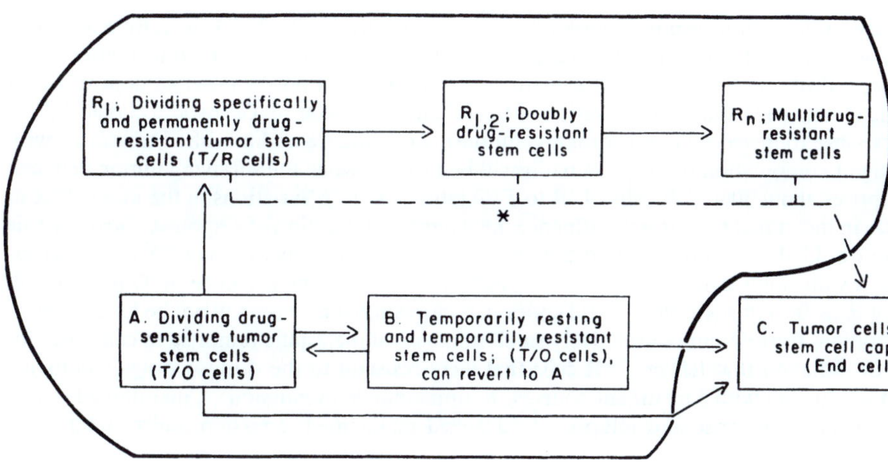

Fig. 2. Tumor stem cell types of major concern in chemotherapy and adjuvant chemotherapy. (1) The origin of different tumor stem cell types is presumed to be $T/O \rightarrow T/R_1 \rightarrow T/R_{1,2} \rightarrow T/R_n$. (2) Initially, in measurable tumors, the nonstem cell compartments C and D may be greater to much greater than the total tumor stem cell burden. Prior to treatment, one may expect the following relative proportions of tumor stem cells in almost any type of neoplasm: $T/O > T/R_1 > T/R_{1,2} > T/R_n$ (if any). Prior to treatment, the ratio of T/R to T/O cells will almost never be as high as 1.0. The nadir in the total tumor stem cell burden achievable by drug A will be reached when the T/A to T/O ratio is about 1.0; when this ratio exceeds 1.0, tumor progression during treatment with drug A will be observed. (3) Chemotherapeutic cure requires the eradication of both T/O und T/R cells. (4) There is an invariable inverse relationship between tumor stem cell burden and curability with chemotherapy, albeit with a wide difference in the total burden curable in different cancers. There is a direct relationship between the total tumor stem cell burden and the probability of the presence of diverse limiting T/R cells

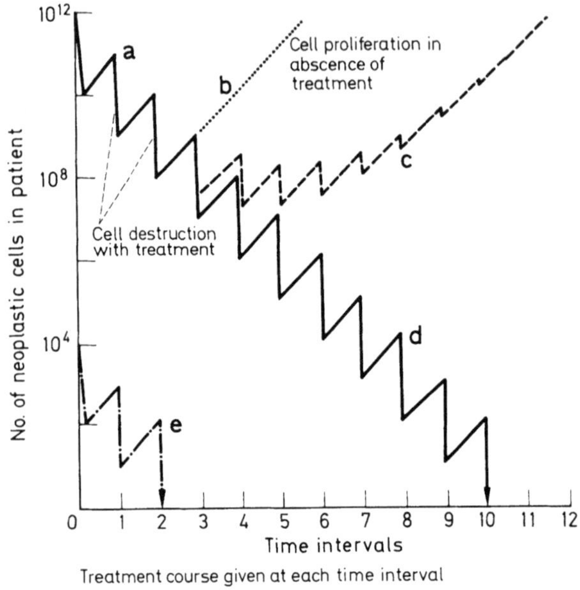

Fig. 3. Idealized time-action response curves for total stem cells (T/O + T/R); equally relevant to chemotherapy alone and adjuvant chemotherapy. *Curve ab,* cessation of treatment after three courses. A second response with the same treatment might or might not be possible depending on the T/R to T/O stem cell ratio at the cessation of treatment and at relapse. *Curve ac,* a classical illustration of response followed by tumor progression during continuing undiminished treatment with the same drug or combination of drugs. A nadir will be reached when the surviving tumor stem cell burden comprises about 50% T/R cells (T/R to T/O ratio = ca. 1.0). Variations in the initial T/R to T/O cell ratio in individual tumors will influence the degree and duration of response. *Curve ad,* this type of curve would almost never be expected on treating individuals bearing, say, 10^9 or greater tumor stem cells with single drugs because of the high probability of the presence of T/R cells with specific resistance. Burkitt's lymphoma and choriocarcinomanoma may or may not be exceptions to this generalization. *Curve e,* cure of relatively small numbers of metastatic tumor stem cells after local surgery or radiation that left no T/R cells that were resistant to the drug or drugs employed. *a,* Remission induction with 3 treatment courses; *b,* unmaintained remission; *c,* maintained remission with decreasing response and relapse; *d,* idealized maintained remission and cellular cure; *e,* adjuvant chemotherapy

search on cancer chemotherapy over the past 25 years have failed to recognize the carryover of many important basic principles.

If someone asked me what features of transplantable neoplasms have been the most helpful in experimental therapeutic research, I would have to answer (1) the relative ease of comparably staging groups of animals - allowing one to determine the phenomena responsible for the invariable inverse relationship between disease advancement and curability with chemotherapy and (2) the fact that the end results of multiarmed experimental therapeutic trials usually are available in 2-3 months instead of 5-10 years. These features are important if one feels the need for some guidance in designing better protocols for treating disseminated human cancers.

Adjuvant Chemotherapy

The use of drugs before or after local treatment to increase the effectiveness of surgery, radiotherapy, or both.

If a neoplastic disease already is widely metastatic, local treatment alone essentially always fails (Fig. 1). It may or may not increase the survival time of surgical failures.

If at diagnosis a measurable primary tumor is present (along with metastatic disease which is not too advanced), chemotherapy alone often fails because it fails to eradicate the T/O and/or the limiting T/R cells in the primary. (See Fig. 2 for definitions of tumor stem cell types that are of major concern in cancer chemotherapy and Fig. 3 and 4 for idealized time-action response curves.)

Adjuvant chemotherapy with single drugs fails if the disseminated disease left after local treatment contains T/R cells that are permanently resistant to the drug employed.

Adjuvant combination chemotherapy often fails when the *metastatic disease* is advanced (e.g., $\geqslant 0.5$ g) and the residual tumor burden after local treatment comprises relatively high proportions of limiting, singly drug-resistant T/R cells and/or smaller proportions of doubly drug-resistant phenotypes.

Adding more and more drugs to an effective combination most assuredly can be counterproductive if this requires reduction in the dose levels or increase in the intervals between delivery of the most effective drug(s) in the combination. (This point has been documented repeatedly in experimental leukemias and solid tumor systems.) When this is done, the multidrug combination may eradicate the T/O cells but fail because the less-effective drugs (or less effectively delivered drugs) did not prevent the overgrowth of T/R cells that are specifically resistant to one or more drugs in the combination. This point has been proven by harvesting neoplasms that regressed and regrew during combination chemotherapy and testing their resistance to each drug in the combination. Such recurring neoplasms are consistently found to be resistant to one or more of the drugs, but usually not to all of the drugs in the combination. The reason for this now seems quite clear.

Analyses of the results of many experimental combination chemotherapy trials carried out in the past have led me to this conclusion: In order for a combination to be maximally effective, it is *critical that the individual doses of all drugs* be selected and matched with respect to (a) the schedule to be used, (b) the growth rate of the neoplasm to be treated, and (c) the expected proportions of limiting T/R cells at different total *tumor cell burdens*. [A rather similar conclusion was reached by Goldie et al. (1982) based on a mathematical development and computer simulations.] Needless to say, these critical variables rarely were taken into account in the design of adjuvant chemotherapy trials carried out over the past 15 years in patients bearing different disseminated cancers.

An Overview (Assigned Subject)

A brief and general survey of theory and the implications of comparative trials in which similarly staged cancer-bearing animals were treated with surgery only, chemotherapy only, or surgery plus chemotherapy. (There is relatively little published data on the effectiveness of radiotherapy plus chemotherapy in experimental cancers.)

In my opinion, the large background of experimental data documenting the *inverse relation* between neoplastic cell burden and curability with chemotherapy alone (albeit with wide variation in the total burden curable in different cancers) is equally pertinent to adjuvant chemotherapy. By now there can be little doubt regarding the consistent direct rela-

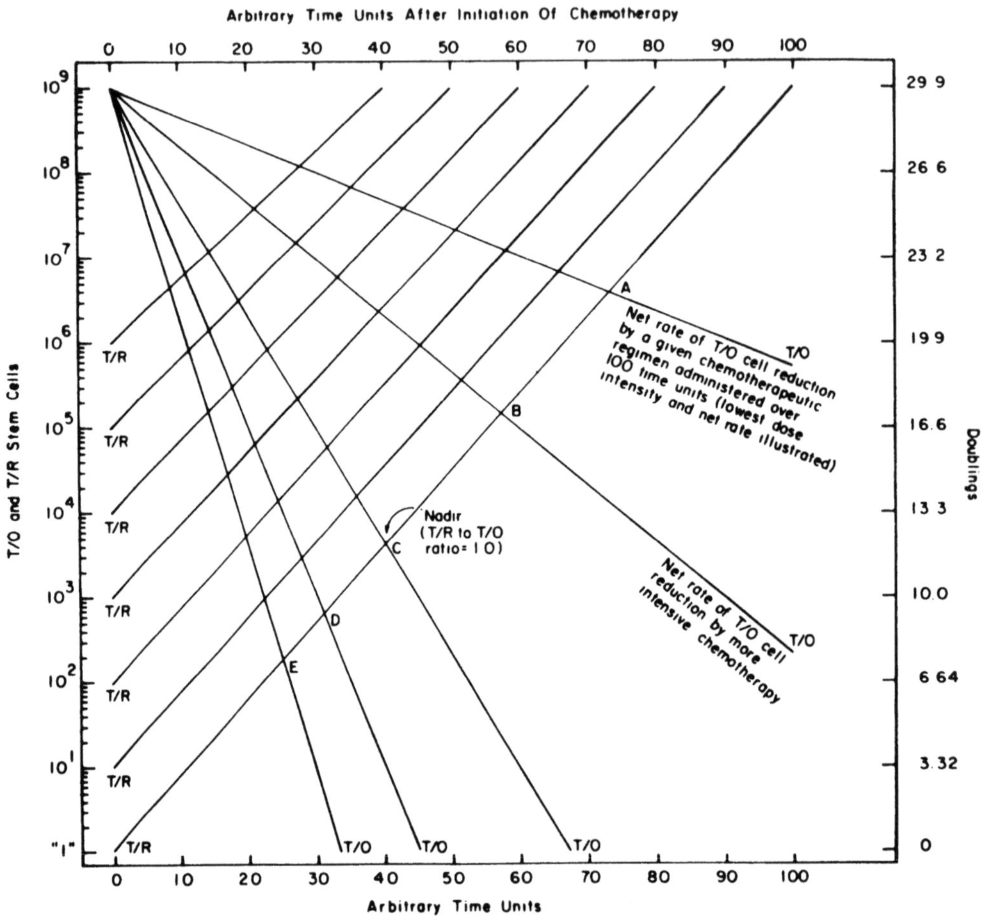

Fig. 4. An idealized nomogram that may help to visualize the influence of (a) the proportion of limiting T/R cells in a neoplasm of a given size, and (b) dose intensity on the degree and duration of response to chemotherapy. (1) In this figure we have illustrated tumors of about the same size (ca. 10^9 total stem cells) comprising widely different proportions of limiting T/R cells.

Designation	Proportion of limiting T/R cells	Classification re: responsiveness to chemotherapy	Potential for cure with combination chemotherapy
(1)	10^8 in 10^9 [a]	Very refractory	Poor
(2)	10^7 in 10^9	Very refractory	Poor
(5)	10^4 in 10^9	Refractory	Fair
(9)	"1" in 10^9	Responsive	Good
(10)	0 in 10^9	Responsive	Good

[a] High probability of the presence of doubling drug-resistant T/R cells.

Note: If the vast majority of the tumor cells were in a primary that could be resected, then surgery + chemotherapy would be expected to be superior to chemotherapy alone in all of these examples, and especially those where the proportion of limiting T/R cells was relatively low. (2) Also illustrated in an idealized manner is the effect of dose intensity on the degree and duration of tumor response.

tion between the total tumor stem cell burden and the probability of the presence of limiting T/R cells. It would be hard to overemphasize the importance of *optimum dosage and delivery of each drug* in a combination of drugs used in an adjuvant setting - in an effort to prevent failures due to overgrowth of limiting T/R cells in metastatic sites.

In this short paper all I can do is tell you what the experimental results I have studied suggest to me regarding questions like these:[1]

1. What phenomena are primarily responsible for cancers being classified as responsible, refractory, or very refractory to chemotherapy?
2. Are the same neoplasms that are responsive and refractory to chemotherapy alone also responsive and refractory to adjuvant chemotherapy - *even when similar burdens of tumor stem cells remain after local treatment?*
3. Why does chemotherapy alone fail when it fails?
4. Why does adjuvant chemotherapy fail when it fails?
5. Why has "surgical adjuvant chemotherapy been a great disappointment after the great rush of enthusiasm that occurred in the early and mid-1970s?" (Carter 1984).
6. Or, has surgical adjuvant chemotherapy already been responsible for saving thousands of human lives (DeVita 1984) - even though we have only begun to design (or redesign) and carry out clinical adjuvant chemotherapy trials taking into account the phenomena that some (including me) believe to be responsible for many past disappointments? (Knowing why one fails does not guarantee future stepwise progress, but it certainly does not hurt the prospects.)
7. Did those of us who were enthusiastic about the prospects of surgical adjuvant chemotherapy in the early and mid-1970s hold out too much hope for magic, or good luck, in *intuitively designed adjuvant chemotherapy protocols?*
8. Having been painfully slow to recognize the critical variables that must be taken into account in the design of optimum combination chemotherapy regimens, should we now reduce or abandon efforts to improve adjuvant chemotherapy protocols? (Certainly not, in my opinion!)

Questions, Deductions, Critical Variables, and Prospects for Improving Control of Disseminated Cancers

The eight questions listed in the "Introduction" seem important to me when I ask: What are the prospects for significantly improving control of disseminated cancers between 1985 and, say, the year 2000?

---

[1] Most of the data and theory that have been influenced by views on these questions have been presented in 177 detailed reports ("Booklets") to the Division of Cancer Treatment of the National Cancer Institute (USA), written between 1974 and February 1985. In aggregate they must weigh a hundred pounds. Some of you who have asked for and received some of these reports have intimated that I must get paid by the pound; this is not true. I believe that one must review old and new data repeatedly, looking for weakness or strength in current concepts

◄ **Fig. 4** *(continued).* The higher the dose intensity, the greater the reduction of *T/O cells* during a given period of treatment and lower the total tumor cell burden at the nadir (T/R to T/O ratio = 1.0). After this nadir is reached, tumor progression will occur during continuing treatment with the same drug or drugs. (3) Inherent in this nomogram is the assumption that all T/O and T/R cells must be eradicated by local treatment, chemotherapy, or both - if cure is to be achieved

Some of these questions are concerned with biological principles, while others have to do with differing opinions. The last two questions were meant to suggest that stepwise progress with adjuvant chemotherapy might have been significantly more rapid in the past if all had realized the critical nature of both the dose level and the interval between delivery of *each drug in a combination* – in attempts to prevent or delay the many adjuvant chemotherapy failures that are due to the overgrowth of limiting T/R cells.

It should be apparent that there is some redundancy in the first four questions posed in the "Introduction". By this I mean if we can (or could) provide reliable answers to question 3 („Why does chemotherapy alone fail when it fails?"), this should shed light on question 1 ("What phenomena are responsible for cancers being classified as responsive, refractory, or very refractory to chemotherapy?"). In may opinion, reliable deductions regarding questions 1 and 3 almost certainly are relevant to question 4 ("Why does adjuvant chemotherapy fail when it fails?").

Only if we can look at the available experimental and clinical data and deduce why adjuvant chemotherapy has failed when it failed can we logically address the "opinion questions," numbers 5–8. (I wish that I could recall the author of this question: "In science, opinions are tolerated only when facts are lacking.") Conceivably, internally consistent deductions regarding questions 1–4 might influence some opinions, reduce the need for endless debate, and result in a reasonably satisfactory basis for future planning. (I do not intend to hold my breath awaiting conceptual unanimity at the 99% level.)

Two Extremely Broad Scientific Questions: Why Does Cancer Chemotherapy Fail When it Fails? What Phenomena Are Primarily Responsible For Cancers Beeing Classified as Responsive, Refractory, or Very Refractory to Chemotherapy?

These are overlapping questions. If we had the answers to one, we probably could deduce the answers to the other. If we had reliable answers to both, we could plan chemotherapeutic regimens more rationally and, I believe, accelerate progress in the treatment of disseminated cancers.

In my opinion, responses to these questions should include discussions of (1) the *biological phenomena* most likely to be responsible for chemotherapeutic failure and (2) *treatment strategies* that might or might not be expected to reduce such failures (depending on the primary cause) when chemotherapy is used alone or in an adjuvant setting.

I imagine that most of us believe that a number of phenomena are responsible for chemotherapeutic failure – in different situations. I also imagine that there is considerable difference of opinion as to the phenomenon that most frequently underlies failure of chemotherapy when used in treatment of some single neoplastic disease or many neoplastic diseases.

I already have thought about and written on both of the above questions – perhaps too often because I find that I am beginning to say some of the same things over and over in somewhat different ways as I examine large bodies of experimental and clinical data (Skipper 1985; Skipper and Schabel 1982, 1984; Skipper and Simpson-Herren 1985).

I admit to past vacillation in my opinion as to the biological phenomenon most frequently responsible for chemotherapeutic failure and for classifications of cancers by chemotherapeutic effect. Is it (a) temporarily resting T/O cells and "growth fraction" differences in different cancers or (b) limiting T/R cells and differences in the proportions of diverse T/R cells in responsive and refractory neoplasms of the same size?

The experimental and clinical data I have examined and reexamined over the past decade have led me to this conclusion: The phenomenon *most frequently* responsible for chemotherapeutic failure is the presence of limiting T/R cells at the initiation of treatment or their emergence during continuing undiminished treatment with the same drug or drugs.

Of the many possible reasons for chemotherapeutic failure this is the only one that satisfactorily accounts for a *very common observation* at both the experimental and clinical levels; namely, objective temporary response followed by tumor progression during continuing undiminished treatment with the same drug or drugs.

This conclusion is abundantly documented in a wide variety of experimental cancers. When neoplastic cells from neoplasms that have regressed and relapsed during treatment with single drugs are passed and retested, they consistently show resistance to the agent that selected them. If such regressions and recurrences are observed during treatment with a combination of drugs, the recurring tumors (on passage and retreatment) are found to be resistant to one or more but not necessarily to all of the drugs in the combination.

It was a paper by Goldie and Coldman (1983) that first led me to think in a different way about why different experimental cancers and different human cancers are classified as responsive, refractory, or very refractory to chemotherapy. Theirs is the first model, of which I am aware, that does not require the assumption that the so-called T/O cells in refractory tumors are more refractory to most or all anticancer drugs *(even when they are dividing)* than the T/O cells in neoplasms that respond well to chemotherapy.

Briefly, their model suggests that (a) "slow" tumor growth often is the result of relatively high rates of tumor stem cell loss due to differentiation or cell death (e.g., when the doubling time far exceeds the average intermitotic time) and (b) tumors in which loss of stem cell capacity occurs with high frequency will have a higher proportion of limiting T/R cells, *at a given size,* than those in which such stem cell loss is infrequent and growth rates are relatively rapid. In this context we might postulate that the *dividing T/O cells* in responsive, moderately refractory, and very refractory neoplasms are equally sensitive to anticancer drugs and that the degree of responsiveness is inversely related to the proportion of limiting T/R cells - or, conversely, the degree of refractoriness to chemotherapy is directly related to the proportion of T/R cells as in Fig. 4.

In a recent examination of the in vitro response to drugs of log phase cultures of tumor cells derived from experimental and human neoplasms, I could find no convincing evidence of marked differences in the sensitivity of the *dividing T/O cells* (Skipper 1985). In fact, in most instances the drug concentrations and the periods of exposure employed were so different that valid comparisons between different tumor cell lines derived from neoplasms that were responsive or refractory to chemotherapy in vivo were not possible.

Some Data and Deductions That Have Influenced the Views Already Expressed

In writing a technical paper, one usually presents observed data and then attempts to suggest what it implies - with appropriate hedging if necessary. In this brief and general survey (overview), I decided to reverse the order and first state my views on the problems and prospects of adjuvant chemotherapy, and follow with a *small sample of data* that I have had the privilege of studying in detail.

In fact, the seeming internal consistency of much diverse data presented and discussed in previous publications already had led me to the views expressed in earlier sections of this review. I will not repeat these observations that seem to me to be compatible in a cross-disciplinary sense.

Table 1. Lewis lung carcinoma; influence of delay in local surgery on the cure rate and survival time of surgical failures (pooled data)

Day of surgery after s.c. implantation of 25-mg tumor fragments	Median survival time (days); cures excluded			% Increase in survival time of surgically treated groups over untreated controls (cures excluded)	Surgical cures	
	After implantation				No./total	%
	Untreated controls[a]	Surgery	After surgery			
2	25	33	31	32	8/ 30	20
3	25	28	25	6	7/ 39	18
4	24	30	26	20	10/ 40	25
6	25	28	22	16	5/ 80	6
Median	25	29	25.5	18	30/199	15
7	30	27	20	0	0/ 50	0
8	27	27	19	0	0/ 18	0
10	29	27	19	0	0/ 48	0
12	29	29	17	0	0/ 60	0
14	27	29	15	7	0/ 40	0
16	30	28	12	0	0/ 28	0
21	32	32	11	0	0/ 10	0

[a] All untreated controls died with large tumors and metastatic disease. The surgical failures died with extensive lung metastases and occasional primary site regrowth

Note: This experimental neoplasm metastasize more rapidly and much more uniformly in individual animals than most transplantable neoplasms we have worked with. At day 7 the primary tumors were about 0.5 g in size

Lewis Lung Carcinoma

Table 1 presents extensive data showing the influence of delay in local surgery on the cure rate and survival time of animals bearing Lewis lung (LL) tumors and associated metastatic disease. If local resection, after s.c. implantation of 25-mg tumor fragments, was delayed for a week or longer, no cures were achieved and no significant increase in the survival time of surgical failures over untreated controls was observed. (In other experiments, bioassays of the lungs and other tissues indicated that by day 7 after implantation essentially all animals were bearing viable lung metastases; some animals had metastatic disease in other sites.) These results show that local surgery was of no benefit after tumor cells had metastasized to vital sites (e.g., the lungs). They also show that removal of the original source of the metastases, after metastasis already had taken place, did not increase survival time, indicating that death resulted from the proliferation of neoplastic cells in metastatic sites. After metastatic tumor cells already were established, subsequent arrival of additional tumor cells was of no consequence. These surgical controls from surgical adjuvant trials seem to show that the LL neoplasm metastasizes more rapidly and uniformly in individual animals than most other transplantable tumors we have studied.

Lewis lung carcinoma is moderately refractory to chemotherapy, depending on the degree of advancement of the solid primary and/or metastatic burden. It responds best to alkylating agents. Table 2 shows the influence of the burden of disseminated LL cells, in the

Table 2. Lewis lung carcinoma; influence of the advancement of disseminated disease (in the absence of a solid primary) and dose level on the cure rate by alkylating agents (pooled data)

Agent	Single dose (mg/kg)	Fraction of the LD_{10}	Percentage of 60-day survivors after single doses on the day indicated		
			Day 2	Day 6	Day 10
Methyl-CCNU	36	1.0	79	71	40
	24	0.67	79	46	6
	12	0.33	26	3	0
Cyclophosphamide	312	1.0	75	84	45
	208	0.67	75	40	6
	103	0.33	80	20	0
CCNU	57	1.0	70	60	10
	38	0.67	20	0	0
	19	0.33	10	0	0

Note: All animals received intravenous inoculation of 10^6 suspended tumor cells on day 0. It is highly unlikely that all or even most of the 10^6 tumor cells had stem cell capacity, but all untreated controls died with extensive lung metastases. The treatment failures also died with extensive lung metastases after varying increases in survival time related to (a) the delay in treatment, and (b) the dose level employed. If the treatment had been delayed for, say, ≥ 15 days, no cures would be expected even with LD_{10} doses of single drugs.

It is reasonable to assume that local surgery plus single-drug treatment will fail in animals bearing primary tumors and high metastatic burdens that contain limiting T/R cells (see Table 3). In such a situation the only apparent way to improve adjuvant chemotherapy is to improve the selection and delivery of non-cross-resistant drugs (combinations) used in conjunction with surgery

absence of a solid primary, and the dose level, on cure rates achieved by alkylating agents. In Table 3 we see the influence of disease advancement on the cure rates achieved by methyl-1-(2-chloroethyl)-3-cyclohexyl-1-nitrosourea (CCNU), cyclophosphamide, and a simultaneous combination of these two alkylating agents. If the primary tumor already was 2 g or greater in size, the best chemotherapy employed in the past provided no complete responses (CRs), much less cures. The results in Fig. 5 show that tumors that regressed and then regrew after two maximum tolerated doses of methyl-CCNU were resistant to this agent when harvested, passed, and retested. In other experiments it was observed that the LL/methyl-CCNU tumor cells were not significantly cross-resistant to cyclophosphamide.

Table 3 provides a comparison of the effectiveness of surgery alone, chemotherapy alone, and surgery + chemotherapy in animals bearing different-sized primary LL tumors and associated metastatic disease. These results indicate that surgery + chemotherapy was consistently superior to single-modality treatment in animals bearing similar tumor cell burdens, and will achieve some cures in animals where essentially no cures are achievable by surgery alone or chemotherapy alone. They also imply that if the disease is too advanced we must expect the adjuvant chemotherapy used to fail – because of the presence of metastatic T/R cells. In order to cure more advanced disease, it would be necessary to improve the combination chemotherapy regimen to be used in conjunction with surgery.

Table 3. Lewis lung carcinoma; a comparison of the influence of advancement of the primary solid tumor and associated metastatic disease on curability by local surgery, chemotherapy, or adjuvant chemotherapy (pooled data)

Days after s.c. implantation of 25-mg tumor fragments	Approximate primary tumor size (g)	% Tumor-free survivors						
		Single modality Rx				Surgery plus:[b]		
		Surgery only	Methyl-CCNU	Cyclophosphamide (CPA)	Methyl-CCNU+CPA	Methyl-CCNU	CPA	Methyl-CCNU+CPA
1-2	<0.1	20-30	60-80	60-100	-	-	-	-
7[a]	0.5	0	34	10	68	40	-	-
12	1.0	0	1	0	24	30	35	70
16	2.0	0	6	0	0	18	15	65
21	≥3	0	0	0	-	0	0	-

[a] At 1 week or greater after s.c. implantation of 25-mg tumor fragments, widespread metastasis was proven by bioassay. Local resection if delayed for 1 week or more never achieved cures and provided little or no increase in the survival time of surgical failures over untreated controls

[b] When surgery was followed by chemotherapy, the interval between was 1-2 days

Note: These results, along with those in Tables 1 and 2 and Fig. 1, indicate that (1) surgery alone fails if the disease is metastatic, (2) chemotherapy alone fails if the primary or metastatic disease is too advanced and contains limiting T/R cells, and (3) surgical adjuvant chemotherapy fails if the metastatic disease is too advanced. The only apparent way to increase the cure rates of more advanced disease is to improve the selection and delivery of combinations of non-cross-resistant drugs used in conjunction with surgery

B16 Melanoma

This experimental neoplasm after many years of transplantation is very refractory to all chemotherapy; it responds best to alkylating agents.

Table 4 lists results obtained in trials where local surgery was delayed for different periods after s.c. implantation of 25-mg tumor fragments. B16 melanoma does not metastasize as rapidly and as uniformly in individual animals as does Lewis lung carcinoma. Although there is a general decrease in cure rate with increasing delay in surgery, it may be seen that in some trials some cures were achieved when surgery was delayed for 2 weeks or longer. In all instances, local surgery significantly increased the median survival time of surgical failures over that observed in concurrent untreated controls.

In Tables 5 and 6 we have listed results of extensive efforts by Griswold and associates to provide quantitative information regarding the B16 stem cell reduction by maximum tolerated doses of methyl-CCNU and cyclophosphamide. Based on the tabulations in Table 6, it would appear that an LD_{10} of methyl-CCNU will eradicate only about 99% of the tumor cells with stem cell capacity. This suggests to me an unusually high proportion of methyl-CCNU-resistant phenotype compared with other experimental neoplasms we have studied. The information in Fig. 6 is consistent with this view.

The data in Table 7 show that a maximum tolerated dose of methyl-CCNU will not cure animals bearing small unmeasurable B16 tumors (25-mg fragments) but will delay tumor appearance and increase survival time. In these comparisons a dose response is apparent.

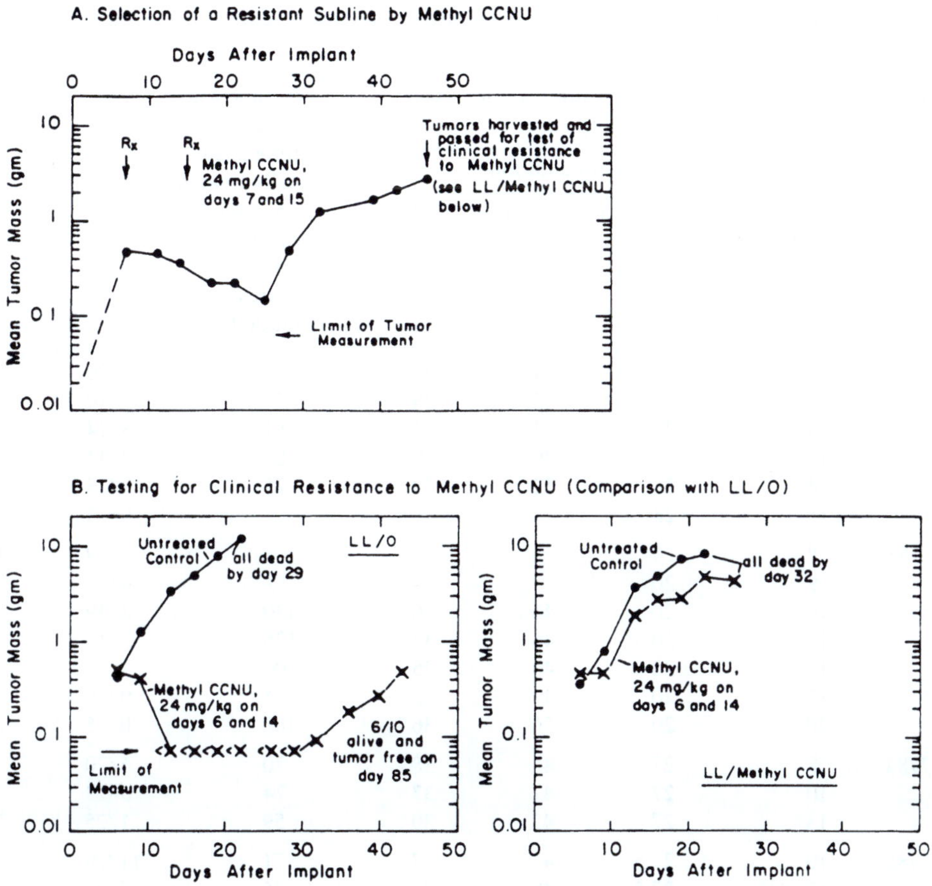

Fig. 5 A, B. Lewis lung carcinoma; selection of a methyl-CCNU-resistant subline by two high doses of methyl-CCNU. **A** The drug-sensitive tumor cell kill doubtlessly was much greater than that seen in the mean tumor mass behavior plotted. Twenty-seven percent (8/20) of the animals in this group were tumor-free on day 46. **B** The first-passage subline of LL tumor selected by methyl-CCNU was markedly resistant to the drug which selected it. The parent line LL/O tested concurrently was quite sensitive; however, the 4/10 relapses presumably would no longer respond to methyl-CCNU but would respond to other classes of drugs which affect LL

Table 8 summarizes the results of trials in which similarly staged animals bearing measurable B16 tumors and associated metastatic disease were treated with methyl-CCNU only, local surgery only, or surgery plus methyl-CCNU.

There are indeed differences in the results and implications of the surgical adjuvant trials carried out in the B16 melanoma and the Lewis lung carcinoma systems. These differences seem important in comparing and interpreting the results of adjuvant chemotherapy results obtained in (a) cancers that are or are not uniformly metastatic at the initiation of treatment and (b) cancers that are responsive, moderately refractory, or very refractory to chemotherapy (Table 9).

Table 4. B16 melanoma; influence of delay in local surgery on the cure rate and survival time of surgical failures

Trial No.	Day of surgery after s.c. implantation of 25-mg tumor fragments	Median survival time (days) excluding cures			% Increase in survival time of surgically treated groups over untreated controls (cures excluded)	Surgical cures	
		After implantation				No./total	%
		Untreated controls	Surgery	After surgery			
7782	8	28	49	41	73	10/20	50
	9	28	45	36	51	7/10	70
	10	28	53	43	81	8/24	33
	11	28	49	38	89	2/11	18
	14	28	52	38	75	0/ 8	0
	15	28	–	–	–	0/ 5	0
7783	8	20	–	–	–	9/ 9	100
	9	20	–	–	–	6/ 7	86
	10	20	46	36	130	8/19	42
	13	20	45	32	125	5/17	29
	15	20	40	25	100	1/ 7	14
	17	20	49	32	145	0/ 9	0
	20	20	56	36	180	0/ 5	0
7784	8	27	46	38	70	6/20	30
	10	27	47	37	74	5/23	22
	13	27	47	30	59	1/25	0
7785	10	27.5	47	37	71	11/29	39
	13	27.5	48	35	75	7/24	29
	15	27.5	65	50	136	2/10	20
	17	27.5	55	38	100	3/ 8	38
	20	27.5	49	29	78	3/11	27

Note: All untreated controls died with large tumors and about 50% exhibited gross metastases; lung metastases were most frequent. Most of the surgical failures exhibited gross metastases at death; about 20% had local recurrences.

B16 melanoma metastasizes less rapidly and less uniformly in individual animals than Lewis lung carcinoma (Table 1). I am somewhat puzzled by the consistent increases in survival time of surgical failures over untreated controls unless large primary tumors contributed to the death of the untreated controls

The above comparison by itself might be misleading, but it becomes more interpretable when considered in the light of all of the data presented in Tables 1–8 and the concepts illustrated in Fig. 1–6.

1. We know that methyl-CCNU is much more effective against similar-sized primary or metastatic burdens of LL than B16 melanoma.
2. We know that LL metastasizes more rapidly and more uniformly in individual animals than B16 melanoma. By the time the primary LL tumor has reached 0.5 g or >, all animals are bearing lung metastases and local surgery provides no cures. On the other

Table 5. B16 melanoma; influence of the size of s.c. inocula of suspended tumor cells on survival time and take rates in untreated animals (pooled data)

Size of s.c. inoculum	Median survival time (days) of dying animals only	Tumor-free survivors	
		No./total	%
10^7	26	0/100	0
10^6	30	2/100	2
10^5	38	2/100	2
10^4	42	12/100	12
10^3	51	35/100	37
10^2	55	67/ 99	68
10^1	(60)	97/100	97
"1"	-	-	-

Note: In these experiments radiation-killed tumor cells were added to the counted inocula to increase the take rate. It is abundantly clear that all of the suspended B16 melanoma cells in the various inocula did not have stem cell capacity. It appears that, on average, only about 0.1%-1% of the tumor cells were viable stem cells. These are untreated control results from trials carried out to determine the relationship between the burden of B16 melanoma stem cells and curability with the drugs that are the most effective against this very refractory experimental neoplasm (see Table 6). The doubling time of the B16 melanoma cells in near exponential phase was between 1 and 2 days

hand, some animals with 0.5- to 4-g primary B16 tumors are not yet bearing metastatic disease and are curable by surgery alone.

3. Is surgery plus methyl-CCNU more effective against B16 melanoma than Lewis lung carcinoma? Not really; surgery + methyl-CCNU provides some cures in animals bearing B16 tumors 3 g or greater because in some animals metastasis has not yet taken place or the metastatic burden is very low and contains no methyl-CCNU-resistant phenotypes. All animals with 3-g or > LL tumors are bearing relatively large burdens of metastatic tumor stem cells, presumably including some that are permanently resistant to tolerated doses of methyl-CCNU.

Adjuvant Chemotherapy Results Obtained in Other Experimental Cancers

This paper already is becoming too long; therefore, I will limit presentation of adjuvant chemotherapeutic results to summaries of results observed in two other experimental neoplasms.

Tables 10 and 11 summarize some results obtained in a colon tumor system (Colon 26) and a mammary tumor system (Mamm 16/C). Both of these neoplasms are refractory to chemotherapy in the sense that cures have rarely been observed in animals bearing measurable primary tumors and associated with metastatic disease.

Table 10 provides data showing the superiority of surgery plus chemotherapy over surgery or chemotherapy in treating animals bearing measurable Colon 26 tumors.

The results in Table 11 provide convincing evidence of the superiority of surgery + Adriamycin over surgery alone or Adriamycin alone in curing animals bearing 0.3-1.0-g Mamm 16/C tumors and associated metastatic disease.

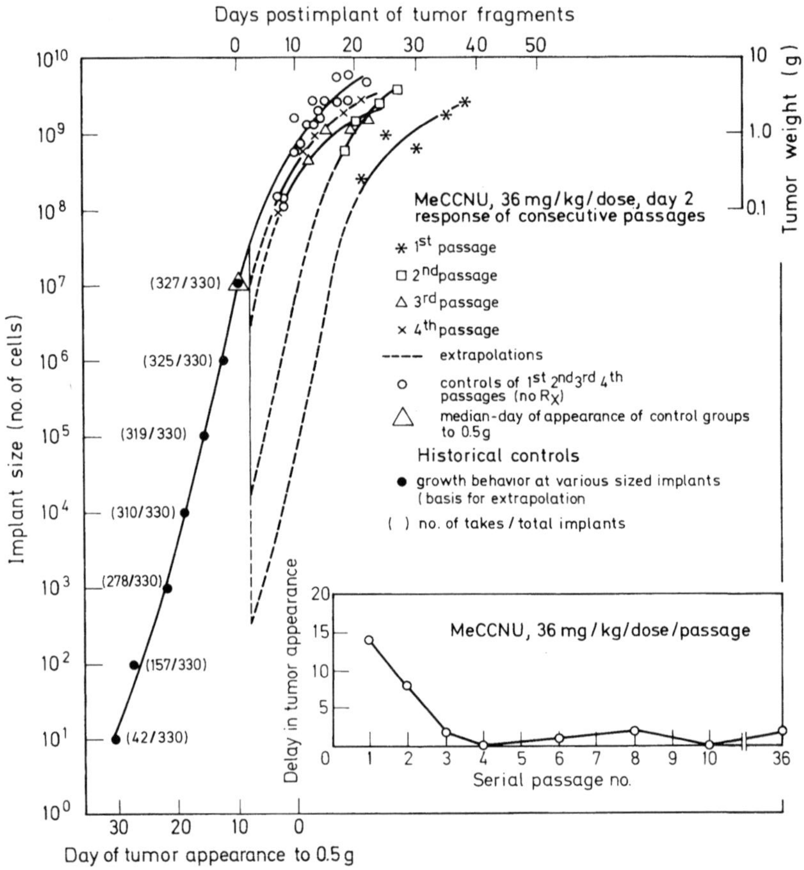

Fig. 6. B16 melanoma; take rate and growth rate in untreated controls and the number of in vivo exposures to methyl-CCNU required to select sublines that are partially or completely resistant to methyl-CCNU. (1) The take rate and growth rate of the parent line of tumor cells are based on extensive pooled data. (2) The number of in vivo exposures (treated passages) required to select sublines that are partially or completely resistant to an LD_{10} of methyl-CCNU was based on the treatment-induced delay in tumor appearance in animals bearing similar burdens of tumor cells that survived 1, 2, 3, 4, or more treated passages - all concurrently compared with the original parent tumor line that never had been exposed to chemotherapy. The extrapolations are made at a growth rate similar to that observed in historical untreated controls. (3) These results imply the following:

B16 tumor cells; 10^7 inoculated s.c. but only about 10^5 with stem cell capacity	Median delay in tumor appearance (days) of groups receiving an LD_{10} of methyl-CCNU compared with untreated controls (parent line)	Estimated tumor stem reduction (logs)
Parent line	14.5	ca. 4
Sublines surviving:		
One Exposure	8	3
Two Exposures	2	1
Three Exposures	0	0.5
Four to ten Exposures	0-1	Insignificant

Table 6. B16; influence of size of s.c. inocula of suspended tumor cells on the survival and survival time of animals treated with methyl-CCNU or cyclophosphamide (data obtained with the L1210 leukemia system for comparison)

Treatment	Single dose (mg/kg)	B16 melanoma (s.c. inoculum)							% Increase in life span of dying animals
		% Tumor-free survivors as influenced by inoculum size							
		10^7	10^6	10^5	10^4	10^3	10^2	10^1	
Methyl-CCNU	40 (LD_{10})	4	0	28	50	-	-	-	12-92
	20	0	0	20	30	40	90	-	14-30
Cyclophosphamide	300 (LD_{10})	0	0	0	0	40	-	-	21-71
	225	0	0	0	0	40	-	-	31-63
None (controls)[a]	-	0	0	3	6	16	52	87	-
		L1210 leukemia (IV inovulum)							
		% Disease-free survivors							
Methyl-CCNU	36	39	80	95	-	-	-	-	> 100
Cyclophosphamide	300	8	30	70	95	-	-	-	> 100
None (controls)[b]	-	0	0	0	0	0	0	5	-

[a] No takes in untreated controls (see Table 5); only about 1% of the inoculated B16 melanoma cells had stem cell capacity on average

[b] Few no takes if the i.v. inoculum is 10^1 or >

Note: Although methyl-CCNU and cyclophosphamide consistently provided significant increases in life span and delays in tumor appearance in animals bearing relatively small burdens of B16 melanoma cells, these data suggest that an LD_{10} of methyl-CCNU did not eradicate much more than 99% of the tumor stem cells. Other assays indicated that a single LD_{10} of methyl-CCNU or cyclophosphamide would reduce the B16 melanoma cell burden by no more than 4 logs and 2.5 logs, respectively (Griswold 1972, 1975; Hill and Stanley 1975). Similar doses of these drugs will cure significant numbers of animals bearing much larger burdens of L1210 (or P388) leukemia stem cells

On the Reason for Failure of CAF to Cure Animals Bearing Measurable Mammary 16/C Tumors

Earlier in this paper I indicated that the data I have studied have led me to conclude that the presence or emergence of limiting T/R cells is the most frequent cause of chemotherapeutic failure – when single drugs or combinations of drugs are used alone or in an adjuvant setting. Years ago it was hoped that intuitively designed regimens of two or three noncross-resistant drugs might prevent failures due to overgrowth of permanently drug-

◀ **Fig. 6** *(continued). Note:* On repeated passage in untreated animals the methyl-CCNU-resistant subline retained its essentially complete resistance to an LD_{10} of methyl-CCNU (Griswold et al. 1981). (4) Conclusion: The proportion of methyl-CCNU-resistant stem cells in the very refractory B16 melanoma is unusually high (ca. 1 in 10^4 to 10^5) compared with the responsive murine leukemias (L1210 or P388) or the moderately refractory Lewis lung carcinoma

Table 7. B16 melanoma; dose response to single doses of methyl-CCNU in animals bearing unmeasurable tumors (treatment 2 days after s.c. implantation of 25-mg tumor fragments); pooled data

No. of experiments	Single dose of methyl-CCNU (mg/kg)	Median delay in appearance of 0.5-g tumors (days)[a]	Median % increase in survival time over untreated controls[b]
21	36 (LD_{10})	15	63
8	30	11	50
28	24	9	26
12	20	5	14
7	16	4	24
4	7-12	0.5	1

[a] Time for tumors to reach 0.5 g; treated minus concurrent untreated controls

[b] Cures were not achieved

Note: Again, methyl-CCNU is the best available drug for treating B16 melanoma, but it will not cure animals bearing unmeasurable tumors (ca. 25 mg in size) nor will it provide good PRs, much less CRs, in animals bearing measurable tumors. The results in Fig. 6 imply that unmeasurable B16 melanoma masses contain relatively high proportions of methyl-CCNU-resistant tumor stem cells

resistant tumor cells. Only recently has it become apparent that it is not that simple or we have not been that lucky. It is critical that dose levels and frequency of administration of *each drug* in a combination be matched so as to minimize the possibility of overgrowth of singly or doubly resistant T/R cells. The results plotted in Fig. 7 illustrate a case in point.

Plot B shows the mass behavior of measurable Mamm 16/C tumors during and after treatment with Adriamycin given at maximum tolerated doses for a q7d (×6) schedule. PRs (partial responses) and CRs were achieved but almost all of the tumors showed progression during the last several doses of Adriamycin. This is almost unequivocal evidence of the overgrowth of Adriamycin-resistant tumor stem cells.

Plot C shows similar regressions and regrowth of Mamm 16/C tumors in animals treated with simultaneous doses of cyclophosphamide, Adriamycin, and 5-fluorouracil (5-FU) (CAF) given q7d (×6). One of the recurring tumors (No. 8) was harvested, passed, and tested for resistance to each of the individual drugs in CAF. It was resistant to Adriamycin but not to cyclophosphamide or 5-FU.[1] Retrospective analyses of the doses of C and A and F used in this trial indicated the probable reason for CAF failure to be overgrowth of Adriamycin-resistant tumor cells. The doses of C and A and F were high enough to eradicate the T/O cells. The doses of C and A and A and F were high enough to prevent overgrowth of the T/F and T/C phenotypes, respectively, but the doses of C and F were too low to prevent overgrowth of the Adriamycin-resistant tumor cells[1] (Skipper and Schabel 1984).

[1] These results were confirmed in a subsequent experiment

Table 8. B16 melanoma; response of similarly staged animals bearing measurable solid tumors and associated metastatic disease to local surgery, methyl-CCNU, and surgery plus methyl-CCNU

Methyl-CCNU (mg/kg/dose)	Schedule days after implant[a]	Approximate primary tumor size (g)	% CRs; methyl-CCNU only	% Increase in life span; excluding cures			% Cures		
				Methyl-CCNU only	Surgery only	Surgery + Methyl-CCNU	Methyl-CCNU only	Surgery only	Surgery + methyl-CCNU
36	9 only	0.5	0	114	121	147	0	20	60
24	9 only		0	35	121	147	0	20	100
54 (toxic)	10 only	1.0	0	47	73	205	0	40	20
36	10 only		0	10	73	135	0	40	30
12	10; qd (× 5)	1.0	0	25	45	82	0	0	30
8	10; qd (× 5)		0	11	45	32	0	0	0
36	13 only	2.0	0	114	116	156	0	20	70
24	13 only		0	51	116	151	0	20	50
24	12; q7d (× 2)	1.8	0	0	41	65	0	0	20
36	16 only	3.5	0	–	19	74	0	0	20
24	16 only		0	–	19	39	0	0	0
36	16 only	3.5	0	19	142	258	0	10	30
24	16 only		0	19	142	160	0	10	30
24	17; q4d (× 4)	4.0	0	0	170	323	0	40	78
20	17; q4d (× 4)		0	27	170	223	0	40	60
16	17; q4d (× 4)		0	0	170	180	0	40	20
		Median	0	22	98	151	0	15 (0–40)	30 (0–100)

[a] All animals received s. c. implants (25-mg tumor fragments) on day 0; all untreated controls died. By day 9 the primary tumors were about 0.5 g in size, on average. There were 100 animals per group in these trials; therefore, small differences in cure rates in single trials should not be considered significant

Note: Surgery + chemotherapy consistently provided greater increase in the survival time of treatment failures than did surgery or chemotherapy alone. It seems apparent that some of the cures in the groups receiving surgery + chemotherapy were surgical cures. The superiority of surgery + methyl-CCNU over surgery alone (when observed) is presumed to be a result of methyl-CCNU eradicating the tumor cells in animals in which very small numbers of B16 melanoma cells remained after surgery (no methyl-CCNU-resistant phenotypes)

Table 9. Lewis lung carcinoma; responses of similarly staged animals bearing measurable solid tumors and associated metastatic disease to local surgery, methyl-CCNU, and surgery plus methyl-CCNU

Tumor system	Approximate primary tumor size (g)	% Curses[a]		
		Methyl-CCNU	Local surgery	Surgery + methyl-CCNU
Lewis lung	<0.1	60–80	–	–
B16	<0.1	0	–	–
Lewis lung	0.5	34	0	40
B16	0.5	0	20	60–100
Lewis lung	1.0	1	0	30
B16	1.0	0	0–40	20– 30
Lewis lung	2.0	6	0	18
B16	2.0	0	0–20	50– 70
Lewis lung	3 or >	0	0	0
B16	3 or >	0	0–40	0– 78

[a] Surgery + methyl-CCNU provided greater increases in survival time in treatment failures, than did surgery or methyl-CCNU alone

Table 10. Colon 26; response of animals bearing 0.5- to 1-g tumors and associated metastatic disease to chemotherapy, surgery, and surgery plus chemotherapy

Chemotherapy	mg/kg/ dose	Chemotherapy schedule (days of Rx)	% CRs[a] (chemotherapy only)	Increase in life span (cures excluded)			% Cures		
				Chemotherapy only	Surgery only	Surgery + chemotherapy	Chemo only	Surgery only	Surgery + chemotherapy
Methyl-CCNU	24	16	60	118	94	–	0	33	100
	24	16	70	218	94	73	0	33	67
	22	16	60	262	171	267	0	27	60
	19	16, 23, and 30	50	210	60	–	0	53	100
	15	15 and 22	10	59	29	39	0	0	67
	15	15, 22, and 29	20	32	29	85	0	0	67
	12	12, 26, and 46	20	183	139	322	0	0	47
	7.3	16, 20, and 24	30	160	171	236	0	27	60
	4	qd 16–24	50	152	171	321	0	27	60
	3.6	qd 12–16, 16–30 and 40–44	10	211	139	356	0	0	67
		Median	40	172	117	252	0	27	67
Methyl-CCNU + 5-FU	20 45	13 13	30	117	36	–	0	47	100
Methyl-CCNU + 5-FU	24 50	14 14	15	168	108	–	0	43	100
Methyl-CCNU + 5-FU	17 15	13 and 20 13 and 20	78	117	36	–	0	47	100
Methyl-CCNU + 5-FU	12 50	13, 20, and 27 13, 20, and 27	80	279	36	–	0	47	100
Methyl-CCNU + 5-FU	10 45	13, 20, 27, and 34 13, 20, 27, and 34	50	149	36	151	0	47	79
		Median	50	149	36	–	0	47	100

[a] Although as high as 80% temporary CRs were observed, chemotherapy provided no cures

Table 11. Mammary 16/C; response of animals bearing 0.3- to 1.0-g tumors and associated metastatic disease to Adriamycin alone, local surgery alone, and surgery plus Adriamycin

Chemotherapy				% Increase in life span (excluding cures)			% Cures		
Adriamycin (mg/kg/dose)	Schedule	%							
		PR+ CR	CR	Adriamycin only	Surgery only	Surgery + Adriamycin	Adriamycin only	Surgery only	Surgery + Adriamycin
14	Single dose	100	70	54	81	131	0	23	68
12	Single dose	80	0	11	8	79	0	0	20
9	Single dose	100	70	41	8	137	0	12	66
8	Single dose	100	40	42	81	117	0	13	45
4	Single dose	0	0	9	16	13	0	11	39
5.8	q7d (×2)	100	80	9	8	96	0	13	47
5.2	q7d (×4)	30	10	26	8	79	0	0	25
			Median	26	8	96	0	12	45

Note: Lung metastases were observed in greater than 75% of animals bearing mammary 16/C tumors in the 0.3- to 1-g size range. Adriamycin is the most effective drug against mam 16/C, but will not cure animals bearing 25- to 50-mg tumors, much less measurable tumors; even 25- to 50-mg tumors contain some Adriamycin-resistant tumor stem cells.

Surgery + Adriamycin is superior to surgery alone in achieving cures of animals bearing 0.3- to 1.0-g mam 16/C tumors and in increasing the survival time of treatment failures

Further analyses suggested that optimally designed regimens of CAF, when given after local surgery, might provide high cure rates in animals bearing measurable tumors (e.g., 0.1-0.5 g) and associated metastatic disease.

In Comparably Staged Groups of Animals Do We See a Relationship Between the Cure Rates Achieved by Surgery Only Versus Surgery Plus Chemotherapy?

As I examined the results of adjuvant chemotherapy trials presented in this report, I thought I saw a trend suggesting a positive answer to the above question. This led to a final tabulation.

Table 12 provides comparisons of cure rates observed in comparably staged groups of animals treated by means of surgery only and surgery plus chemotherapy. The concurrent comparisons in randomized groups are listed in decreasing order of the cure rates achieved by surgery only.

My interpretations of these comparisons are indicated in the brief comments in Table 12.

◀ **Table 10** *(continued). Note:* These are internally controlled multiarmed trials in which there were 15 animals/group. Surgery was carried out 1-2 days before chemotherapy when both treatment modalities were used. This neoplasm does not metastasize as rapidly or uniformly as Lewis lung carcinoma. These results leave little doubt regarding the superiority of surgery + chemotherapy in animals bearing 0.5- to 1.0-g tumors and 50% or more of the animals bearing metastatic disease. On the other hand, had all of the animals been bearing, say, 0.5-g or > of metastatic disease, neither surgery nor surgery plus the chemotherapy used would be expected to achieve cures

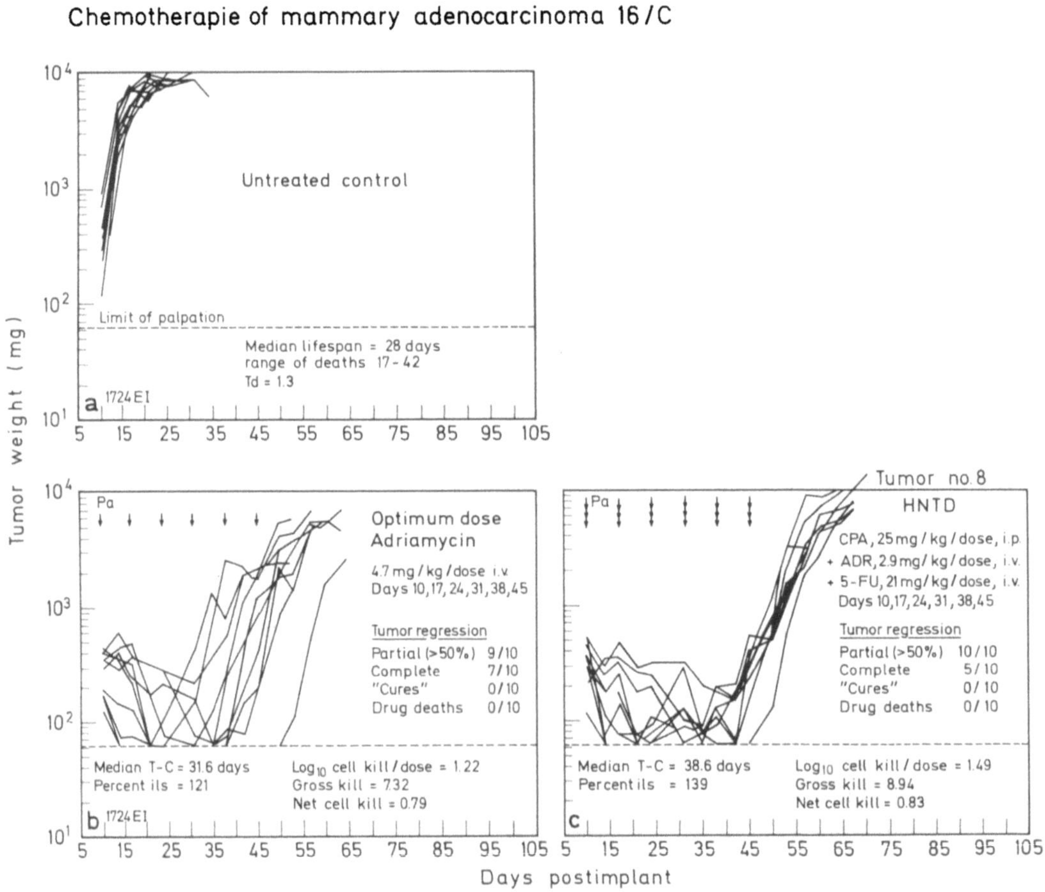

Fig. 7 a–c. Mammary adenocarcinoma 16/C; temporary PRs and CRs followed by regrowth during repetitive weekly doses of Adriamycin and CAF. **a** Untreated controls; **b** adriamycin, 4.7 mg/kg per dose, q7d (×6) starting on day 10 (note regrowth during courses 3, 4, 5, and 6); **c** CAF, q7d (×6), starting on day 10 (note regrowth during courses 5 and 6). Tumor no. 8 was harvested, passed to other animals, and tested for resistance to each drug in the combination. The tests showed the tumor cell population (in tumor no. 8) to be resistant to adriamycin but not to cyclophosphamide or 5-FU

Summary

Brief responses to some questions posed in the text might serve as a summary to this paper. These responses represent my own opinions which have been influenced by (a) experimental and clinical results obtained with single drugs and combination chemotherapy used alone and in an adjuvant setting and (b) what I consider to be current theory that has evolved from years of basic and pragmatic research by many investigators.

1. What phenomena are responsible for different cancers being classified as responsive, refractory, or very refractory to chemotherapy?
   Presumably there are several, but differing proportions of limiting T/R cells – in neoplastic cell populations of the same size – appears to be *the most frequent single phenomenon* underlying such classifications (see Figs. 2–4). (The relative proportions of

Table 12. In comparably staged groups of tumor-bearing animals do we see a relationship between the cure rate achievable by surgery only versus surgery-chemotherapy?

Tumor	% Cures in comparably staged groups		Comment
	Surgery only	Surgery plus chemotherapy	All animals were bearing measurable solid tumors at the time of treatment. Some animals were bearing metastatic disease at the time of treatment; others were not (excepting Lewis lung carcinoma)
Lewis Lung carcinoma	0	40	No cures with surgery only; decreasing cure rate with increasing delay in surgery + chemotherapy and increasing metastatic burden
	0	30, 35, 70[a]	
	0	18, 45, 65	
	0	0, 0	
B16 melanoma	40	78, 60, 20[b]	A seeming direct relationship between the cure rate achieved by surgery versus surgery + chemotherapy. This neoplasm is very refractory to chemotherapy and it does not metastasize as uniformly in individual animals as LL. Presumably many of the surgery + chemotherapy cures were, in fact, surgical cures
	40	30	
	20	60, 100	
	20	70, 50	
	10	30, 30	
	0	30, 0	
	0	20	
	0	20, 0	
Colon tumor 26	53	100	A seeming relationship between the cure rate achieved with surgery and surgery + chemotherapy. This neoplasm is very refractory to chemotherapy; cures are not achieved by chemotherapy alone if the primary tumors are already measurable. Presumably many of the cures achieved by surgery + chemotherapy were, in fact, surgical cures, but this does not detract from the value of chemotherapy in animals bearing tumor stem cells beyond the reach of local surgery
	47	100[c]	
	47	100[c]	
	47	100[c]	
	47	100[c]	
	33	79[c]	
	33	100	
	27	67	
	27	60	
	27	60	
	0	60	
	0	67	
	0	67	
	0	47	
Mammary 16/C	23	68[d]	A possible relationship between the cure rate achieved with surgery and surgery + chemotherapy. It is likely that the failure of surgery + Adriamycin (when it failed) was due to metastatic Adriamycin-resistant tumor stem cells
	12	66	
	12	47 Median	
	12	45 46	
	12	39	
	0	25	

[a] Treatment with methyl-CCNU, CPA, or methyl-CCNU + CPA (respectively)
[b] Different dose levels of methyl-CCNU
[c] Treated with methyl-CCNU + 5-FU; other groups treated with methyl-CCNU only
[d] All groups were treated with Adriamycin

Note: In some instances primary site regrowth was observed in surgical failures. In such a situation adjuvant chemotherapy must eradicate the residual local as well as widely disseminated tumor stem cells. In the future I intend to examine the results of other sets of experimental adjuvant chemotherapy results in a similar manner

limiting T/R cells with specific and permanent resistance to many or most drugs appear to be in this order: very refractory > moderately refractory > responsive neoplastic diseases.)

2. Are the same neoplasms that are responsive and refractory to chemotherapy alone also responsive and refractory to adjuvant chemotherapy – even when similar burdens of tumor stem cells remain after local treatment? The answer to this question seems to be "yes," at least with respect to the data I have examined.
3. Why does chemotherapy alone fail when it fails? The answer to this question seems consistent with the response to question 1. The most frequent cause of chemotherapeutic failure is the presence of limiting T/R cells that overgrow during continuing undiminished treatment with the same durg or drugs.
4. Why does adjuvant chemotherapy fail when it fails? For much the same basic reason underlying failure of chemotherapy alone, i.e., excessive numbers of limiting T/R cells remaining after local treatment. Surgical adjuvant chemotherapy is consistently superior to surgery alone, but fails to increase the cure rate if the limiting T/R cells in the metastatic burden cannot be eradicated by the particular chemotherapeutic regimen employed.
5. Why has "surgical adjuvant chemotherapy been a great disappointment after the great rush of enthusiasm that occurred in the early and mid-1970s?" This is an opinion that might (or might not) be tempered by questions 6, 7, and 8.
6. Or, has surgical adjuvant chemotherapy already been responsible for saving thousands of human lives – even though we have only begun to design (or resign) and carry out clinical adjuvant chemotherapy trials taking into account phenomena that some believe to be responsible for many past disappointments? I share the opinions implied in this question for reasons given in the text of this paper.
7. Did those of us who were enthusiastic about the prospects of adjuvant chemotherapy in the early and mid-1970s hold out too much hope for good luck or magic in *intuitively designed* adjuvant chemotherapy protocols?
   To be frank, I cannot recall precisely what I thought 10–15 years ago except that I was convinced of this broad biological principle: there is an invariable inverse relationship between the neoplastic stem cell burden and curability with chemotherapy, albeit with widely different total burdens curable in different neoplastic diseases. For this reason I thought the long-term prospects of adjuvant chemotherapy were good if we could continually improve the designs of combination chemotherapy regimens as had been done in the treatment of some leukemias and lymphomas. In this expectation I may have been wrong. In many instances the stepwise changes in chemotherapy protocols for use in an adjuvant setting were not stepwise improvements.
8. Having been painfully slow to recognize the critical variables that must be taken into account in the design of optimum combination chemotherapy regimens, should we now reduce or abandon efforts to improve adjuvant chemotherapy protocols? Certainly not, in my opinion.

Acknowledgment. The experimental adjuvant chemotherapy trials considered in this paper were carried out at the Southern Research Institute between 1965 and 1980 with support from the Division of Cancer Treatment, National Cancer Institute.

The experimental work with the different experimental neoplasms was planned and supervised by the following: Lewis lung carcinoma, Mayo, Laster, and Schabel; B16 melanoma, Griswold, Dykes, and associates; Colon 26, Corbett, Griswold, and associates; and Mammary 16/C, Corbett, Griswold, and associates.

Much more information regarding these systems may be found in numerous publications by the above. I am grateful to all of them for the privilege of examining their raw data in the context of this particular paper (in 1985).

I do wish to acknowledge the conceptual contributions of those who first advocated treatment of disseminated cancers with adjuvant chemotherapy: Martin, Cole, Fisher, Nissen-Meyer, and a few others. As I recall, their advocacy in the 1950s and 1960s did not immediately increase their popularity among some groups.

References

Carter SK (1984) Adjuvant chemotherapy in osteogenic sarcoma: the triumph that isn't. J Clin Oncol 2: 147-148

DeVita VT (1984) Opening comments: only if you believe in magic. In: Salmon SE, Jones SE (eds) Adjuvant therapy of cancer IV. Grune and Stratton, Orlanda, pp 3-16

Goldie JH, Coldman AJ (1983) Quantitative model for multiple levels of drug resistance in clinical tumors. Cancer Treat Rep 67: 923-931

Goldie JH, Coldman AJ, Gudauskas GA (1982) Rationale for the use of alternating non-cross-resistant chemotherapy. Cancer Treat Rep 66: 439-449

Griswold DP Jr (1972) Consideration of the subcutaneously implanted B16 malanoma as a screening model for potential anticancer agents. Cancer Chemother Rep 3: 315-324

Griswold DP Jr (1975) The potential for murine tumor models in surgical adjuvant chemotherapy. Cancer Chemother Rep 5: 187-204

Griswold DP Jr, Schabel FM Jr, Corbett TH, Dykes DJ (1981) Concepts for controlling drug-resistant tumor cells. In: Fidler IF, White RJ (eds) Design of models for testing cancer therapeutic agents. Van Nostrand Reinhold, New York, pp 215-224

Hill RP, Stanley JA (1975) The response of hypoxic B16 melanoma cells to in vivo treatment with chemotherapeutic agents. Cancer Res 35: 1147-1153

Skipper HE (to be published) Laboratory models: some historical perspective. Cancer Treat Rep (Special Symposium Issue: Laboratory models and clinical cancer)

Skipper HE (1985) What phenomena are primarily responsible for cancers being classified as responsive, refractory or very refractory to chemotherapy? Southern Research Institute, Birmingham, pp 201-203 (Booklet 2)

Skipper HE, Schabel FM Jr (1982) Quantitative and cytokinetic studies in experimental tumor systems. In: Holland JF, Frei E III (eds) Cancer medicine, 2nd edn. Lea and Febinger, Philadelphia, pp 663-685

Skipper HE, Schabel FM Jr (1984) Tumor stem cell heterogeneity: implications with respect to classification of cancers by chemotherapeutic effect. Cancer Treat Rep 68: 43-61

Skipper HE, Simpson-Herren L (1985) Relationship between tumor stem cell heterogeneity and responsiveness to chemotherapy. In: DeVita VT, Hellman J, Rosenberg SA (eds) Important advances in oncology 1985. Lippincott, Philadelphia, pp 63-77

Theoretical Considerations Regarding the Early Use of Adjuvant Chemotherapy

J. H. Goldie and A. J. Coldman

Division of Medical Oncology, Cancer Control Agency of British Columbia,
600 West 10th Avenue, Vancouver, B. C., V5Z 4E6, Canada

Introduction

There is now a large amount of information from both clinical and experimental studies that indicate that there is a strong inverse correlation between tumor mass and potential curability by drugs (Skipper 1978; DeVita 1983). All other things being equal small tumor burdens will be much more susceptible to drug-induced cure than will large. This has been shown for a wide variety of transplanted rodent tumors and, as well, the same inference can be clearly made from clinical observation. For those disseminated malignancies for which curative chemotherapy is available, there appear to be no exceptions to the general statement that patients presenting with a significantly lower tumor burden are much more likely to achieve cure than those patients with the same histological disease who present with very extensive tumor burdens (Frei 1982). The extension of these concepts into the area of the treatment of more refractory groups of malignancies yields the conclusion that it may be possible to achieve drug-induced cures in patients with microscopic tumor burdens whereas the same disease at an advanced stage would be incurable. It is this hypothesis which has now become the underlying rationale for the utilization of so-called adjuvant chemotherapy.

This appreciation of the relationship between tumor burden and curability has not always been the basis for the application of adjuvant drug treatment. In the early studies of this approach it was felt by some investigators that the important role of chemotherapy was to sterilize any cancer cells that might be dislodged from the primary tumor during surgical manipulation. Although such dislodgment of viable cancer cells may well occur during surgery, it is now appreciated that a far more serious problem limiting the curative potential of surgery is the presence of distant metastases which have arisen long before surgical extirpation of the primary tumor.

In this review we well discuss some of the phenomena that might contribute toward more effective utilization of chemotherapy. In particular we well be interested in those factors that would argue for the utilization of chemotherapy at the earliest time feasible, i. e., even before removal of the primary lesion is undertaken.

Factors Favoring the Curability of Small Tumors as Compared with Large Tumors

A number of processes have been postulated to be of importance in rendering small or microscopic tumor burdens more susceptible to drug-induced cure as compared with large ones. A phenomenon that is frequently invoked is the overall growth kinetics of the neoplasm (Steel and Lamerton 1968). In most experimental solid tumors it is possible to

Recent Results in Cancer Research. Vol 103

show that during the earlier stages of growth a tumor mass tends to have different growth kinetics than when it reaches some limiting size. During these early stages the overall doubling time of the neoplasm tends to be shorter and the growth fraction and labeling index will be larger. These factors appear to correlate with increased drug sensitivity assuming of course that the cells within the tumor are inherently susceptible to the drugs that are being utilized in treatment. It is unlikely, however, that kinetics on their own provide a comprehensive explanation of the relationship between tumor mass and curability, either in experimental or clinical situations.

For one thing, curability in a number of experimental tumors appears to diminish significantly over tumor size ranges, where there has been no measurable alteration in growth kinetics (Skipper et al. 1964). Moreover, a purely kinetic explanation of treatment failure would imply that prolonged application of the same drug treatment should result in higher cure rates. In general this is not observed.

As well, correlation between drug curability and growth kinetics in clinical malignancies is only an approximate one (Schackney et al. 1978). There is a tendency toward poor responsiveness to drugs among more slowly growing neoplasms but there can be substantial overlap among individual tumors and indeed classes of tumors with respect to their degrees of drug sensitivity and their inherent cell kinetic properties. And finally tumors that become unambiguously resistant to drug treatment usually do not display any obvious change in their growth kinetic properties.

Nonetheless, the correlation that does tend to exist between more rapid growth kinetics and increased drug sensitivity is likely valid up to some point and may at least reflect on properties of the neoplasm that do render it more susceptible to chemotherapeutic action. An unanswered question at the present time is whether deliberately altering the growth kinetics of a tumor (i.e., by the stimulation of growth in a hormone-dependent neoplasm) can in fact predictably increase the drug sensitivity of the tumor. If such effects could be demonstrated than this would have important implications for the use and timing of adjuvant chemotherapy.

Another issue which may be of considerable importance and which appears to relate to the kinetic properties of metastatic disease is the phenomenon which has been described by Simpson-Herren et al. (1976) (see also the discussion by Fisher et al. volume). It has been observed in a number of experimental neoplasms (but not all) that removal of the primary growth by surgery is followed by a measurable (though temporary) increase in growth rate in the metastatic foci. It would seem reasonable to imagine that this process on its own, unhindered by therapy, might be purely detrimental to the host. Abrogation of this phenomenon by early postoperative (and, perhaps, preoperative) chemotherapy might reduce some potentially disadvantageous effects of surgical removal of the primary.

The biological basis of this "postsurgery growth spurt" is unknown nor is it clear whether it occurs during the surgical treatment of clinical disease. It clearly may be an important aspect in relation to perioperative chemotherapy, and requires further detailed investigations.

In experimental neoplasms and from what can be more indirectly inferred from the behavior of clinical disorders, it would appear that another very important consideration with respect to the utilization of chemotherapy is the issue of the presence of drug-resistant cells within the tumor (Skipper 1978).

We have previously published mathematical and computer-based models of the process of spontaneous mutations to drug resistance (Goldie and Coldman 1979; Coldman and Goldie 1983), and have examined some of the inferences of these phenomena with respect to optimality criteria for cancer chemotherapy. These inferences will be examined in more detail with particular reference to the question of optimal timing of adjuvant drug treatment.

The Relationship Between Tumor Size and Drug Resistance

If one assumes a random and spontaneous origin of drug-resistant phenotypes within a tumor then it is possible to develop an explicit relationship between tumor size and potential curability. If we assume that the absence of any drug-resistant cells constitutes the minimum conditions for curability then the probability of zero-resistant cells becomes equivalent to the probability of cure. This is of course assuming that sufficient courses of therapy are administered to eradicate all of the drug-sensitive cells within the tumor.

As we have previously reported (Goldie and Coldman 1979) this analysis predicts a steep quantitative relationship between tumor size and likelihood of cure. The probability of zero-resistant cells follows a Poisson distribution and generates a characteristic sigmoid shape curve where probability of cure is plotted against log tumor size.

A feature of this relationship which is not intuitively obvious is the steepness with which the probability of cure declines as tumor burden increases. For any given value of the mutation rate this probability will go from a high to a low level within an increase in tumor burden of less than two logs (approximately equal to six volume doublings). Depending upon the growth rate of the neoplasm, this shift in probability of cure could occur over a relatively short period and over a period representing a small fraction of the total biological history of the tumor.

For tumors which are growing relatively rapidly then elapsed periods of time as short as 30 days might be expected to have definite impact on prognosis with respect to chemotherapy. Self-evidently, if the growth rate of the neoplasm is very slow, i. e., a volume doubling time of 100 days, then delays in the institution of chemotherapy would be expected on average to have relatively little impact.

This steep relationship between tumor size and curability has been confirmed for a number of transplanted rodent tumors. It is not known at the present time whether this relationship is as steep in clinical neoplasms and therefore the question as to the advantage gained from the very early use of chemotherapy must still be considered an open one.

It is clear that the early use of adjuvant chemotherapy will likely have significant impact on survival if (1) the doubling time of the subclinical malignancy is relatively short and (2) a significant proportion of individual patients have tumor volumes that are distributed across the steep portion of the probability of cure curve. If the tumor growth is very rapid and if a high proportion of patients have tumor burdens in the critical mass region then one would predict that moving the time forward for the initiation of chemotherapy by periods as short as 3–4 weeks might generate improved results sufficient to be detected in appropriate clinical trials.

In contrast, however, we may have situations where the doubling time of the tumor is quite long and where the distribution of tumor mass is over a very wide range, with relatively few cases falling over the critical transition size. Then one would expect that pre- or perioperative chemotherapy in these cases would not generate detectable improvements in therapeutic end results, compared with adjuvant chemotherapy given up to 1 month postsurgery.

Therefore from the point of view of the drug resistance model the utility of neoadjuvant chemotherapy is going to be heavily influenced by the actual growth rate of the tumor and the frequency distribution of subclinical tumor burdens.

One might reasonably infer that malignancies that tend to show rapid doubling times at the advanced stage will almost certainly be characterized by similar or greater rapid growth rates in the subclinical stage. With more slowly growing tumors or tumors that show a great deal of heterogeneity with respect to growth rates at the advanced stage then inferences about the behavior of the neoplasm during the subclinical phase have to be more tentative. It is generally assumed, by analogy with many experimental tumors, that tumor growth rates will be more rapid during the subclinical or microscopic period. This need not be true for every type of tumor.

Likewise, we usually have no accurate means at present for estimating directly the range of distribution of subclinical tumor burdens. This can be estimated indirectly by examining the times to relapse in patients who receive locoregional therapy alone. Sources of error in these estimates are of course significant.

Clonogenic Cell Mass and Curability

In the minimal drug resistance model initially proposed the simplifying assumption that all cells in the tumor had clonogenic or stem cell capacity was made. This is clearly a significant oversimplification for the situation pertaining to spontaneous clinical neoplasms. Considerable evidence from a variety of sources would indicate that in most categories of clinical malignancy only a very small proportion of the morphologically malignant cells have the biological potential for unlimited growth (Bush and Hill 1975; Buick and Mackillop 1981; Bush et al. 1982). Most of the cells that can be seen within a neoplasm have a proliferative potential analogous to the differentiating cells within a normal cell renewal system. The cells may have the ability to undergo several sequential divisions and to generate a large number of progeny but ultimately these cells become functionally terminally differentiated and cease division permanently.

The so-called stem cell model of tumor biology has a number of implications for the expected behavior of clinical tumors undergoing treatment by chemotherapy. Of particular relevance to our discussion here is the fact that (1) the true tumor burden as measured by actual clonogenic cells may be much smaller the gross tumor burden as measured by all of the constituent cells of the neoplasm and (2) 100% eradication of all of the viable cells in the tumor may not be necessary for there to be an appreciable chance of cure. Since there will be a significant probability that at division the progeny of the clonogenic cell will lose stem cell capacity then for tumor burdens of less than 100 clonogenic cells there will be a nonnegligible possibility that all of the constituent stem cells will become extinct. This probability rises steeply as one deals with ever smaller clonogenic cell burdens.

Our analysis of the situation that occurs when one assumes renewal probabilities of less than one for the stem cell compartment are of some interest here (Goldie and Coldman 1983). Essentially, the same steep relationship between tumor burden and potential curability is found to exist even when one goes to the more complex dynamic model. The steep relationship between clonogenic cell burden and tumor size persists and again the time frame over which this curability changes is related to the doubling time of the clonogenic cells. The predictions of this more complex model with respect to the potential advantages of pre- or perioperative chemotherapy are essentially the same as those for the minimal model. As with the minimal model the impact of early chemotherapy is going to be heavily influenced by the actual doubling time of the clonogenic cells (i. e., their renewal probability) and the distribution of clonogenic cell mass in sample populations of patients. Where the doubling times are short and where the distribution of clonogenic cell burden is in the critical size range then again one would predict for a significant impact by the use of early adjuvant chemotherapy. A slow-growing neoplasm that exhibited a wide range of size distribution would be predicted to be significantly less influenced by the early use of chemotherapy.

Conclusions

Aside from the effect of cell kinetics and the presence of drug resistance there are other factors that might argue for the use of preoperative chemotherapy. In certain types of neoplasms the use of chemotherapy prior to surgery may permit the application of less radical surgery, such as limb-sparing procedures in the treatment of hard and soft tissue sarcomas. In some protocols the use of preoperative chemotherapy has been utilized to assess the drug sensitivity of the primary neoplasm and on that basis to select appropriate drugs for the application of the chemotherapy during the postoperative period.

If we consider the phenomenon of mutations to drug resistance then the impact of early chemotherapy will be maximized under conditions where the growth rate of the neoplasm is rapid and where the distribution of subclinical tumor burdens is over a relatively narrow range. It the relatively narrow range of subclinical burdens is close to the theoretical probability of cure curve for a given chemotherapeutic regimen then relatively short delays in the institution of treatment will permit significant numbers of patients to move from a condition of high probability to low probability of cure. The period over which this will occur will as mentioned previously be dictated by the actual volume-doubling time of the tumor when it is in this size range.

In this context we would like to point out that the importance of eliminating undue delays in the institution of adjuvant chemotherapy has not always been fully appreciated. During the earlier years of breast adjuvant chemotherapy, we can recall many anecdotal instances where the adjuvant treatment was delayed for up to 3 months following surgery. Except for the most slowly growing tumor this would clearly appear to represent an unacceptable delay. With the recognition that time is an important consideration there has been a steady trend toward reductions in time delays for the institution of postoperative chemotherapy. This should be reflected in trends toward better end results with adjuvant programs, but, also, from the perspective of drug resistance, will make it increasingly difficult to demonstrate statistically significant differences between pre- and postoperative chemotherapy. In the extreme case would the drug resistance model predict significant differences between an adjuvant program that was started 24 h before surgery compared with one that was started 24 h after? The answer is obviously not, though other factors might come into play to determine which of the approaches was better, i. e., drug toxicity, logistical feasibility, etc.

It may be therefore that not every type of clinical malignancy will benefit from or require the urgent application of chemotherapy as the primary treatment mode. There would appear, however, to be no way to resolve this issue other than by carrying out the appropriate prospective studies. One can say, providing the chemotherapeutic regimens did not compromise the ability to deliver locoregional treatment or result in its delay, they should have no potential for adversely affecting the impact of adjuvant chemotherapy and may well in specific classes of tumor have the potential for measurably increasing long-term survival and cure rates.

References

Buick RN, Mackillop WJ (1981) Measurement of self-renewal in culture of clonogenic cells from human ovarian carcinoma. Br J Cancer 44: 349-355

Bush RS, Hill RP (1975) Biologic discussion augmenting radiation effects in model systems. Laryngoscope 85: 1119-1133

Bush RS, DeBoer G, Hill RP (1982) Long term survival with gynecological cancer. In: Stoll BA (ed) Prolonged arrest of cancer. Wiley, New York, pp 27-58

Coldman AJ, Goldie JH (1983) A model for the resistance of tumor cells to cancer chemotherapeutic agents. Math Biosci 65: 291-307

DeVita VT Jr (1983) The relationship between tumor mass and resistance to chemotherapy. Cancer 51: 1209-1220

Frei E III (1982) The National Cancer Chemotherapy Program. Science 217: 600-606

Goldie JH, Coldman AJ (1979) A mathematic model for relating the drug sensitivity of tumors to their spontaneous mutation rate. Cancer Treat Rep 63: 1727-1733

Goldie JH, Coldman AJ (1983) Quantitative model for multiple levels of drug resistance in clinical tumors. Cancer Treat Rep 67: 923-931

Schackney SE, McCormack GW, Cuchural GJ Jr (1978) Growth rate patterns of solid tumors and their relation to responsiveness to therapy: an analytical review. Ann Intern Med 89: 107-121

Simpson-Herren L, Sanford AH, Holmquist JP (1976) Effects of surgery on the cell kinetics of residual tumor. Cancer Treat Rep 60: 1749-1760

Skipper HE (1978) Cancer chemotherapy. I: Reasons for success and failure of treatment of murine leukemias with the drugs now employed treating human leukemias. University Microfilms, Ann Arbor

Skipper HE, Schabel FM Jr, Wilcox WS (1964) Experimental evaluation of potential anticancer agents. XII: On the criteria and kinetics associated with "curability" of experimental leukemia. Cancer Chemother Rep 35: 1-111

Steel GG, Lamerton LF (1968) Cell population kinetics and chemotherapy. Natl Cancer Inst Monogr 30: 29-50

Experimental Preoperative Chemotherapy

L. M. van Putten*

Radiobiological Institute TNO, P.O. Box 5815, 2280 HV, Rijswijk, The Netherlands

Introduction

Preoperative adjuvant chemotherapy in experimental tumors is not new; more than 25 years ago Brock (1959) described the advantage of preoperative chemotherapy in a rat tumor (Table 1). The results were quite impressive, especially if these tumors were more than 10 g at the time of treatment. Not all tumors show a similar response and for that reason it is useful to compare different models. This report describes the response of three mouse tumors to adjuvant chemotherapy with cyclophosphamide given before or after surgical removal of the primary tumor. In order to obtain early metastasis, the tumors were inoculated into the mouse foot pad (Mulder et al. 1983). The basic data on the three tumors are presented in Table 2.

Lewis Lung Tumor

The Lewis lung tumor is sensitive to chemotherapy with cyclophosphamide only when it is small (see Table 3). Subcutaneously inoculated tumors may be cured in 92% of the cases if treatment is given early, and in foot pad tumors in 33%. In contrast, neither cure nor growth delay is observed after chemotherapy if the tumor is first allowed to grow in either site until it is just palpable. In the adjuvant situation treatment is given before or after surgical removal of the primary tumor in the foot pad at the time when surgery without chemotherapy leads to about 90% of mice dying from pulmonary metastasis. As shown in

Table 1. Data of Brock (1959) on early versus late adjuvant chemotherapy of Shay chloroleukemia in the rat

		% Cures
A	Cyclophosphamide[a] without surgery	30
B	Surgery without chemotherapy	10
C	Cyclophosphamide during and 1 day after surgery	50
D	Cyclophosphamide 8 and 7 days before surgery	90

[a] Groups A, C, and D received two doses of 30 mg/kg

* The following also participated in this study: J. H. Mulder, J. de Ruiter, P. Lelieveld, M. B. Edelstein, T. F. C. Gerritsen, R. J. F. Middeldorp, T. Smink, and L. K. J. Idsenga

Recent Results in Cancer Research. Vol 103

Table 2. Basic data on three tumors studied

Name	Lewis lung	Mammary carcinoma 2661	Osteosarcoma
Host	C57B1/Ka	CBA/Rij	{CBA × C57B1}F1
Origin	Philadelphia 1951	Rijswijk 1961	Rijswijk 1957
Passage	> 100	> 80	78-84
Flank inoculum	10^6	10^6	10^6
Foot pad inoculum	10^5	10^5	10^5
Metastasis to lung	100%	73%	100%
Metastasis to lymph nodes	12%	93%	43%
Cyclophosphamide Dose (mg/kg)	100	200	50 or 100

Table 3. The relation between tumor size and response to cyclophosphamide

Localization and size at time of therapy	Growth delay and percentage cures	
	Lewis lung	Mammary 2661
Subcutaneous flank tumor		
Day 3	16 days 92%[a]	18 days 7%[a]
Day 10	4 days 0%	12 days 4%
Foot pad tumor		
Day 3	3 days 33%[a]	36 days 13%[a]
Day 10	1 day 0%	10 days 0%

On day 3, tumors are not yet palpable; on day 10 all of them are
Results are averages from pooled data of several experiments; each group contained at least 50 mice
[a] Significant difference with untreated control ($P < 0.05$)

Table 4. The effect of treatment with cyclophosphamide in combination with surgery

Chemotherapy	*Lewis lung*			*Mammary 2661*		
	ILS	ICR	*P*	ILS	ICR	*P*
Before surgery	15 days	25%	< 0.001	10 days	20%	< 0.01
After surgery	30 days	40%	< 0.001	20 days	0%	NS

ILS, increase in life span of nonsurvivors; *ICR*, increase in cure rate
Foot pad tumors were amputated at 3-4 weeks after implantation. Around 90% of surgical control mice dies (all from lung metastases). Chemotherapy was given 2-3 days before or 2-3 days after surgery. The data represent the results of pooled experiments totaling 60-110 mice per treatment group

Table 4, the treatment before surgery is less effective than after surgery. There are not only fewer cures, the growth delay of the relapsing tumors is also shorter. A possible explanation of this phenomenon may be found in the lower growth rate of measurable metastases from Lewis lung tumor (Simpson-Herren et al. 1976). This would be associated with a lower sensitivity of resting cells to drug treatment. A mechanism of this type has not been reported for other tumor models and since a more rapid growth of metastases after removal of the primary tumor is not a frequent phenomenon in clinical oncology, this model is probably not representative of the majority of human tumors.

Mammary Carcinoma 2661

This tumor is less sensitive to cyclophosphamide. Treatment of mice 3 days after inoculation of this tumor subcutaneously in the flank or in the foot pad causes no cures (see Table 3) but a major prolongation of survival by 18 days for the flank tumors and 36 days for the foot pad tumors. If treatment is delayed until the tumors are palpable, the growth delay is reduced to 12 and 10 days, respectively. In the adjuvant situation there is an increase in cure rate only if treatment is given before surgery, as indicated in Table 4.

If the experimental mice are subdivided according to size of the foot pad tumor, it appears that the benefit of adjuvant therapy is seen mainly among the mice with large foot pad tumors. In this group where there are no survivors without adjuvant therapy, a major effect of adjuvant cyclophosphamide is noted in contrast to the group with small primary tumors where mortality was unaffected by adjuvant treatment. Postoperative chemotherapy led to an increase in survival time but not in cure rate. The possible counterpart of this model in clinical disease is a strong argument in favor of exploring in patients the effects of chemotherapy before surgery.

Osteosarcoma C22LR

This tumor is very sensitive to cyclophosphamide chemotherapy; large flank tumors may be cured with two doses of 250 mg/kg cyclophosphamide. Adjuvant therapy at a dose of 50 mg/kg was without effect, but a dose of 100 mg/kg caused an increase in cure rate that is quite independent of the time of administration (see Table 5). It is obviously a manifestation of a different type of response from the two other tumors, but at present we have no explanation for it. The advantage of early treatment is that it offers the possibility of cur-

Table 5. Effect of adjuvant therapy on osteosarcoma

Dose, 50 mg/kg cyclophosphamide	Survivors/treated	
Control	4/24	
Treated day 3	4/24	
Dose, 100 mg/kg cyclophosphamide	**Survivors/treated**	
Control	15/45	33%
Treated day −3	29/38	76%
Treated day +3	28/38	74%
Treated day +10	19/24	79%

Table 6. Frequency of lymph node and lung metastasis of osteosarcoma 18 days after inoculation into the testicle

Treatment	Number of mice	% Mice with metastasis in	
		Lymph nodes	Lung
None	200	77	7
Cyclophosphamide, 250 mg/kg	44	16[a]	30[a]
CCNU, 75 mg/kg	35	0[b]	26[b]

[a] $P<0.01$; [b] $P<0.001$ for difference with controls
CCNU, 1-(-2-chloroethyl)-3-cyclohexyl-1-nitrosourea

ing those animals that have a small tumor burden. Apparently 70% of mice have low burdens before surgery. It is puzzling to be forced to conclude that is still the case 10 days after surgery.

In 1975 we reported on the paradoxical effect of treating tumors with chemotherapy after inoculation into the testicle (van Putten et al. 1975). The reason for the experimental approach was a report that tumor inoculation at this site in hamsters would rapidly lead to lymph node metastases (Rivenzon and Comisel 1967). This was confirmed by our findings in mice and in some cases we observed lymph node metastases even if we amputated the injected testicle 2 h after tumor cell inoculation, a finding that suggests a very rapid transport of some of the inoculated cells into the lymphatics. If high-dose chemotherapy was given 2 h after tumor cell inoculation into the testicle, a paradoxical effect of increased lung metastases was noted (Table 6). This occurred notwithstanding the high effectiveness of the cytostatic agents used.

The chemotherapy resulted frequently in the complete cure of the testicular tumor, but the administration shortly after inoculation of the tumor cells was apparently ineffective against the migrating cells in the lymph nodes and actually enhanced the spread of the tumor to the lung. It is likely that tumors that are not sensitive to cyclophosphamide or nitrosoureas would under similar conditions show an even more marked spread than this sensitive tumor.

Conclusions

The experimental approach of adjuvant chemotherapy for rodent tumors is very different from the clinical studies. The advantage of experimental studies with transplantable tumors in rodents is the possibility to reproduce similar types of disease in the model systems opening the road to comparison of different types of treatment, e.g., preoperative versus postoperative adjuvant therapy. This is a major advantage since it permits us to obtain valid conclusions on mechanisms after the observation of a small number of similar animals carrying a somewhat uniform disease. There are, however, technical disadvantages in most of the experimental metastasis systems. In models, as in man, metastasis is not a uniformly reproducible process. After inoculation of tumor in mice there is a marked heterogeneity in the time of appearance of metastases. For that reason we make use of tumor inoculation into the foot pad of the mouse, since growth at this location leads to early - and therefore to relatively uniform - metastases. That is, uniform compared with what we would obtain after tumor cell inoculation at other sites, but nevertheless far more heterogeneous than in a group of patients in a clinical trial. If the time of removal of the primary tumor is selected so that we have 10%–30% of animals without metastases, there are apt to be 20%–40% of animals that have metastases of a size comparable to clearly manifest disease in man. It is obvious that we have to be very critical when attempting to draw conclusions that may be valid for human disease.

But that is not the only limitation. Usually we study metastatic disease in laboratory animals in a single tumor or a few different tumors. Remember that this implies collecting information on the equivalent of one or a few human patients. Of course the information is much more detailed and it may be very suggestive if the few animal tumors studies are shown to respond in a similar way. That is not the case and we can only conclude that the experiments suggest that it is worth the effort to test preoperative adjuvant chemotherapy in patients.

References

Brock N (1959) Neue experimentelle Ergebnisse mit *N*-Lost-Phosphamidestern. Strahlentherapie 41: 347–354

Mulder JH, de Ruiter J, Edelstein MB, Gerritsen TFC, van Putten LM (1983) Model studies in adjuvant chemotherapy. Cancer Treat Rep 67: 45–50

Rivenzon A, Comisel V (1967) Experimental model for the induction of tumoral lymph node metastasis in hamsters. Experientia 23: 756

Simpson-Herren L, Sanford AH, Holmquist JP (1976) Effects of surgery on the cell kinetics of residual tumor. Cancer Treat Rep 60: 1749–1760

Van Putten LM, Kram LKJ, van Dierendonck HHC, Smink T, Fazy M (1975) Enhancement by drugs of metastatic lung nodule formation after intravenous tumour cell injection. Int J Cancer 15: 588–595

Implications of Certain Cell Kinetic and Biological Parameters for Preoperative Chemotherapy

B. T. Hill

Laboratory of Cellular Chemotherapy, Imperial Cancer Research Fund, Lincoln's Inn Fields, London WC2A 3PX, Great Britain

Introduction

The object of cancer chemotherapy is to do the maximum damage to the tumor and the minimum damage to the patient. This objective is most likely to be achieved when full-dose intensive drug combinations are administered on a frequent intermittent schedule at the earliest opportunity in the course of the disease. Experimental evidence to support this contention has been available for over a decade from laboratory studies and certainly provides a sound basis for preoperative chemotherapy. Those data will be reviewed briefly in this presentation, with emphasis on their demonstrated and potential clinical relevance.

Factors Contributing to the Failures of Chemotherapy

The emergence of drug-resistant tumor cells during cancer chemotherapy constitutes a formidable obstacle to achieving long-term remission or cure (Goldie et al. 1982). In addressing this problem Goldie and Coldman (1979) developed a somatic mutation model and have shown that the number and proportion of resistant cells will increase during the lifetime of the tumor and that advanced tumors will contain substantial proportions of such cells. Therefore cancer chemotherapy fails because we do not exploit its true potential and use it *before* drug resistance has developed. The main reason for this is our inability, using currently available methods of investigations, to detect most tumors clinically until they are at least two-thirds of the way through their life span. This point is illustrated in Fig. 1, which shows the relationship between the number of population doublings of the tumor, the increase in tumor cell number and weight during development, the level of clinical detection, and the death of the patient. Because most human tumors are late or advanced at the time of presentation, failure to "cure" patients using chemotherapy alone should not be unexpected. This also applies to the detection of metastatic disease so that it is quite likely, for a patient with an apparently "local" tumor, to have many undetectable distant micrometastases. Indeed, this micrometastatic spread, which has occurred prior to local-regional therapy, is responsible for the vast majority of treatment failures and therefore must be the main target for adjuvant chemotherapy.

In clinical studies altered drug responses have been observed not only following repeated courses of chemotherapy but also after radiotherapy (Holland et al. 1980; Price and Hill 1981 a; Wolf and Chretien 1981; Paulson et al. 1982; Young et al. 1982). The decrease in response rate of previously irradiated patients to subsequent chemotherapy is generally considered to be associated predominantly with impairment of the blood supply to the tumor from radiation-induced vascular fibrosis. However, even in those patients with recur-

Recent Results in Cancer Research. Vol 103

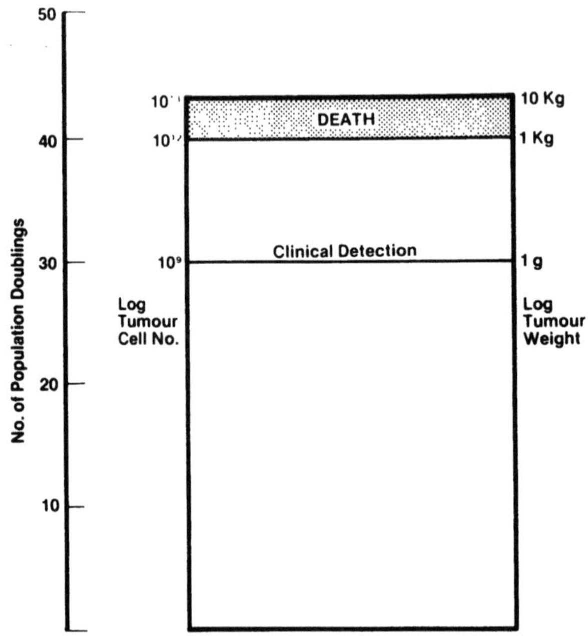

Fig. 1. The relationship between the number of population doublings and the increase in cell number and weight during the development of the tumor, its clinical detection, and the death of the patient. Current methods of investigation enable the tumor to be detected when about 1 g of tumor is present and the tumor is already at least two-thirds of the way through its life span

rent disease, objective responses to chemotherapy frequently occur in slightly less than half of those treated, for example, in head and neck cancer (Price and Hill 1981a; Wolf and Chretien 1981); *but* the duration of response is generally short, so that postradiation chemotherapy has had no significant impact on survival (Hill et al. 1984b). This initial, but unsustained, response argues against markedly impaired drug delivery to previously irradiated tumors and implies involvement of cellular phenomena. For example, it is possible that radiation treatment may have induced drug-resistance and thus subsequent drug treatment could provide a positive selection pressure for these resistant tumor cells, resulting in the growth of a drug-resistant population.

We have used continuous human tumor cells lines in culture to determine whether fractionated X-irradiation in vitro leads to altered drug responses (Hill and Bellamy 1984; Hill et al. 1984c, 1985). Since most radiotherapy is administered in fractionated dosage, we adopted this procedure in our experimental studies, selecting as the radiation dose per fraction that required to produce a 1-log cell kill. The total dose administered approximated that used clinically, according to the histological tumor type under investigation. Initially we used a cell line derived from a human squamous cell carcinoma of the tongue, but more recently have extended our investigations to include human lines derived from a breast carcinoma (MCF-7) and a transitional cell carcinoma of the bladder (RT 112). We first established that the growth characteristics of the radiation-pretreated sublines and the parental lines were comparable. Then we derived dose-response curves for a number of standard antitumor agents, assessing survival by clonogenic assays following a 24-h drug exposure and compared results obtained with the parental and radiation-pretreated sublines. Three general patterns of response have been identified after this fractionated-radiation pretreatment: (1) enhanced sensitivity, for example, to 5-fluorouracil, hydroxyurea, and cisplatin, (2) unaltered responses, to Adriamycin and methotrexate, and (3) marked resistance, to etoposide and vincristine.

This first experimental demonstration that exposure to fractionated radiation induces cellular changes associated with altered drug responses may have major implications for the combined modality approach to the treatment of human cancers. It may prove beneficial in planning adjuvant therapies to use certain drugs *before* radiation treatment, while other drugs may prove particularly valuable *after* radiotherapy. This latter point links well with the idea stressed by DeVita (1983) of the potential importance of highlighting any collateral sensitivity as one approach to overcoming drug resistance.

Evidence in Favor of Adjuvant Chemotherapy

In attempting to design optimal adjuvant chemotherapy a number of factors needed to be considered. There is well-established evidence, derived from laboratory studies with tumor-bearing animals, that: (1) chemotherapy is more effective against small rather than large advanced tumors (Skipper et al. 1965; Schabel 1977) and (2) rapidly proliferating cell populations are most sensitive to the cytotoxic effects of drugs (Bruce et al. 1966; Valeriote and van Putten 1975). To assess the value of these observations in providing a basis for the optimal clinical usage of chemotherapy, various groups have attempted to determine whether comparable evidence is available from experimental data derived from human tumors.

Cell Kinetic Characteristics of Human "Solid" Tumors

The size of the tumor and the rate at which it grows is influenced by a number of kinetic parameters including: the rate of cell production, the growth fraction, the cycle times of proliferating cells, the extent of cell loss and cell turnover, and the size of the stem cell population. These factors have been extensively reviewed (Hill 1978 a) so that only certain aspects will be highlighted here.

Tumor Crowth Rate. A characteristic feature of the growth of a tumor is a progressive increase in cell number. In experimental model systems, such as in vitro cultures of tumor cells or ascitic animal tumors or transplantable leukemias, a constant relationship between cell division and time is observed and these tumor cells are described as growing exponentially. In many "solid" tumors in animals, however, while the logarithm of tumor cell number increases linearly with time during the earliest period of a tumor's development, as the tumor mass increases, its inner and outer regions become subject to different physiological conditions which affect its pattern of growth; there is a tendency for the growth rate to slow and the growth curve is then described by a Gompertzian function. For most human "solid" tumors, where estimations of tumor growths are of necessity restricted to a short period near the end of their life span (see Fig. 1), any attempt to use these measurements as a basis for future treatment planning must be approached cautiously. With this and the other limitations discussed earlier in some detail (Hill 1978 a), it is hardly surprising that the quoted doubling times of human "solid" tumors range from 66 h to 600 days. Such figures reflect at the very least a marked heterogeneity not only between different tumors evaluated but even within the same tumor when multiple biopsies

Table 1. Estimations of traditional cell cycle kinetic parameters on human "solid" tumors. (Hill 1978a)

Tumor parameter	Range of values quoted
Doubling time	66h to 600 days
Fraction of dividing cells	30% to 100%
Intermitotic time	14h to 9 days
Duration of the S phase	12h to 30h
Growth fraction	20% to 70%
Cell loss factor	30% to 99%

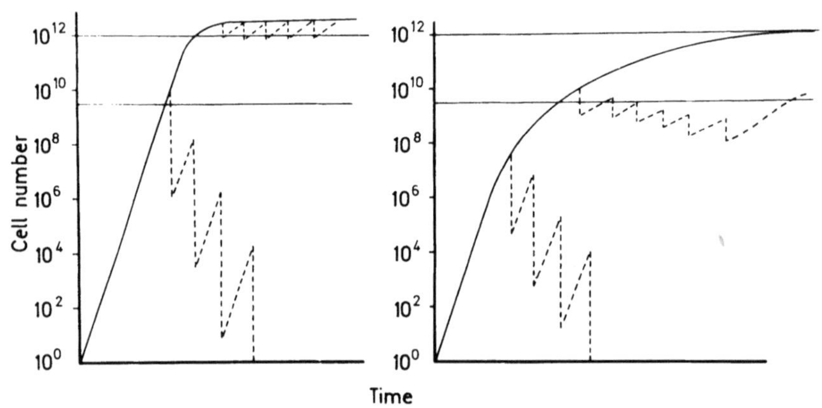

Fig. 2. Schematic representation of fractional cell kills in rapidly growing and slowly growing human tumors. (Schackney et al. 1978)

have been tested. Heterogeneity is also evident in most of the other kinetic parameters which various workers have attempted to quantitate in these clinically detectable advanced tumors (Table 1). However, the rate at which tumors grow is likely to influence the effectiveness of chemotherapy. Skipper's fractional cell kill hypothesis (Skipper et al. 1965), indicating that effectiveness of drug treatment increases with decreasing number of tumor cells, was derived from the exponentially growing murine L1210 leukemia, although it has subsequently been validated in other animal tumors (Wilcox et al. 1965; Schabel 1977). For many human "solid" tumors with a slower growth rate it can be seen from Fig. 2 that the necessity for early treatment is even more vital if cure is to be achieved. Figure 2 also shows that treatment effective at the time of clinical detection for exponentially growing tumors, since fractional cell kills were large, would not result in cure if the tumors exhibited Gompertzian type growth. Under these conditions, with small fractional cell kills, at best a shallow response would be followed by early recurrence. Only treatment of subclinical disease, producing larger fractional cell kills, may in these circumstances lead to cure (Shackney et al. 1978). These data clearly argue in favor of adjuvant chemotherapy *but* also stress the importance of achieving large fractional cell kills. Therefore, although experimental studies have shown that chemotherapy ist more effective against small rather than large tumors, this should *not* be taken to imply that micrometastatic tumors can be killed readily by "low-dose" chemotherapy. Furthermore, depending on the time when metastasis occurred, these tumors may already contain drug-resistant clones.

Proliferating and Nonproliferating Cell Populations. Although it has been shown experimentally that rapidly proliferating cells are more sensitive to the cytotoxic effects of antitumor drugs than nonproliferating cells, optimal adjuvant chemotherapy must also eradicate these nonproliferating tumor cells. In vitro studies comparing tumor cells in the plateau or stationary growth phase with those growing exponentially have demonstrated that most antitumor drugs exert selective toxicity against proliferating cells, as reviewed earlier (Hill and Baserga 1975; Hill 1982). Only a few drugs have been identified as either equally toxic to proliferating and "resting" cells or preferentially toxic to the "resting" population; these include cisplatin, mitomycin C, and the nitrosoureas. However, there are conflicting opinions as to the validity of these model test systems and the questionable relationship of such artificially produced "nonproliferating" populations to those in human "solid" tumors. So while it might be an advantage to include one or more of these drugs in combinations used as adjuvant chemotherapy, it would not necessarily overcome or reduce the problem imposed by noncycling tumor cells. It should be remembered that heterogeneity exists even among nonproliferating cells; some are sterile or end cells, but others remain only temporarily at rest. For example, in "solid" tumors some nonproliferating cells arrested by lack of nutrients or toxicity are destined to die, while others may recover when the supply of nutrients improves, perhaps following partial destruction of the tumor by therapy. A partial depletion of the proliferating population, for example by chemotherapy, also may trigger both normal and malignant resting cells back into cycle. In addition, in cells proceeding slowly or discontinuously through the cycle, their traverse may be speeded up by an appropriate stimulus. In certain normal tissues, the resting or nonproliferating population represents an essential element in homeostasis, which may also be the case in certain malignant tumors. Thus a knowledge of the size of all these subpopulations of the utmost importance before any significance can be attached to the frequently quoted values for the "proliferative or growth fraction" in human tumors. Published information provides a range of values from 20% to 70% for the "growth fraction" of "solid" tumors (Steel 1977) and any correlations between growth rate and growth fraction are very tenuous. Available data do not support the widely held beliefs, frequently cited, that: a low "growth fraction" is a consistent phenomenon of "slow-

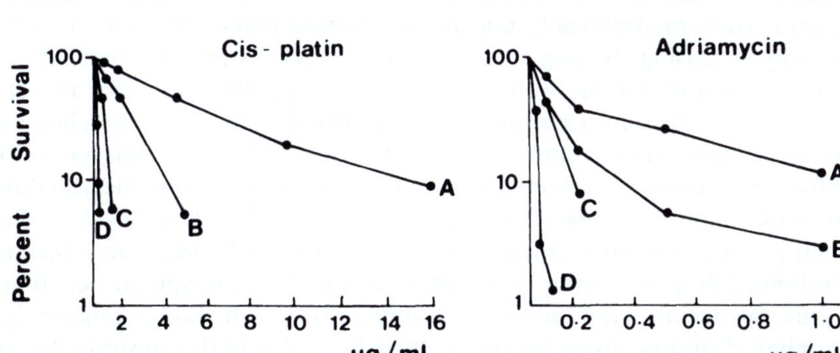

Fig. 3. Dose-response curves for human ovarian carcinoma cells treated in vitro with cisplatinum or Adriamycin over a range of exposure times. Increased tumor cell kill results from either increasing drug concentration or prolongin exposure durations. *A*, 1hr; *B*, 6hr; *C*, 18 hr; *D*, continuous exposure

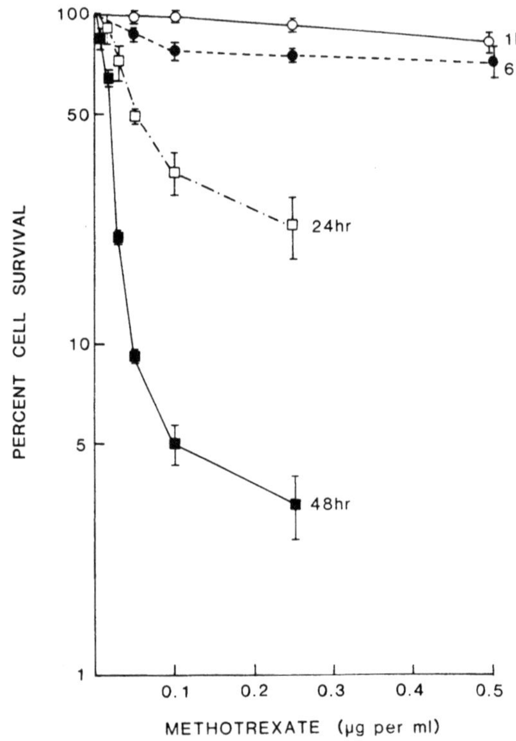

Fig. 4. Survival of human neuroblastoma cells from line CHP 100, estimated by colony-forming assays, after treatment in vitro with a range of methotrexate concentrations for variable exposure times of 1-48 h. The cytotoxic effects of methotrexate are related more to duration of exposure than to drug concentration. (Hill and Price 1982)

growing" tumors, or that tumors with low "growth fractions" will *not* be susceptible to chemotherapy.

An alternative approach toward destroying or reducing these nonproliferating tumor cell populations, which might be exploited clinically, involves the time-dependent cytotoxic effects known to be exerted by antitumor drugs. Initial laboratory evidence, subsequently confirmed clinically, is available showing that increased tumor cell kill results, not only by increasing the drug concentration, but also by prolonging the duration of drug exposure (see, for example, Hill and Price 1982; Rupniak et al. 1983; Hill et al. 1984d). Figures 3-5 provide some experimental data derived from studies with human biopsy material or human tumor continuous cell lines which illustrate this point. Therefore more effective adjuvant chemotherapy may result from modifying the scheduling of currently available antitumor drugs. Any tumor cells triggered back into cycle, induced to speed up their proliferation rates, or those with longer cell cycle times, may become vulnerable to prolonged drug exposures. However, for any definite therapeutic benefit to accrue normal tissue damage must not increase concomitantly. It is therefore of major significance that a number of studies, discussed below, have been able to demonstrate that selective toxicity against the tumor can indeed be achieved using a 24-h drug exposure duration.

Stem Cells. Tumor heterogeneity is also evident when considering the proliferative potential of cells within any population. The large majority of cells are characterized by a re-

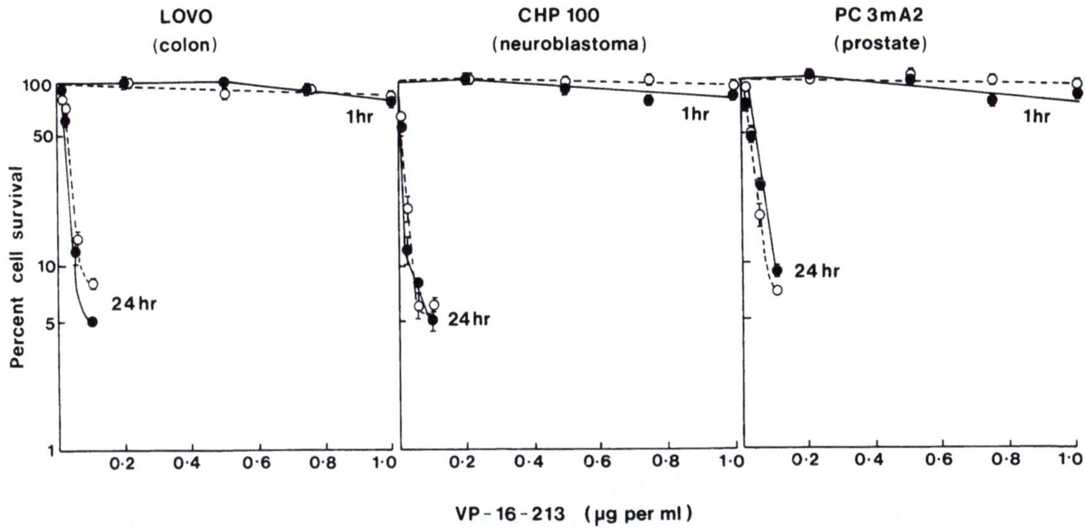

Fig. 5. Dose-response curves for a series of continuous human tumor cell lines derived from different histological tumor types treated in vitro with VP-16-213 (etoposide) for 1 or 24 h. Survival was assessed using either the Courtenay assay (•) or the Hamburger and Salmon assay (o). Duration of exposure is an important determinant of etoposide-induced cytotoxicity under these experimental conditions

stricted capacity for proliferation and will die after a limited number of divisions. A small proportion of cells, the so-called "end" cells, are terminally differentiated and incapable of further division, whilst another small fraction of the total population have the capacity for unlimited proliferation and are termed "stem" cells. It is the stem cell population which is responsible for maintaining the integrity and continued survival of any particular cell population (Mc Culloch and Till 1971). The existence of stem cells in normal tissues is well established, with those in bone marrow and intestinal crypts being particularly well characterized (Carnie et al. 1976), and evidence of malignant stem cells is gradually accruing (Bruce et al. 1966; Hamburger and Salmon 1977; Buick 1984; Thomson et al. 1984).

Malignant stem cells are the most important cells in tumors since they are capable of self-renewal and migration, so allowing growth of the primary and initiation of distant metastases; their growth properties must be characterized and their susceptibility to drugs established. Definitive evidence of the presence of stem cells in human "solid" tumors has awaited the establishment of reliable assay procedures. Significant advances have been made in the past decade with the development of in vitro agar colony-forming systems (reviewed by Hill 1983), which support the growth of a variety of human tumor cells derived directly from patients' biopsy samples. Results from these studies indicate that the proportion of clonogenic cells in tumors is low, being of the order of 0.01%-1%. It remains to be established whether this methodology provides accurate quantitation of the total tumor stem cell population, but it seems likely that the lower values of 0.01% may well be improved upon by identifying more favorable and perhaps unique growth environments in vitro for cells derived from tumors of different histological types. Current investigations aimed at defining the responses of these clonogenic tumor cell populations, derived from human tumor biopsies, have generally resulted in accurate definition of their patterns of drug resistance, by correlation with lack of clinical responses, with a predictive accuracy of approximately 90% (von Hoff et al. 1981; Mann et al. 1982; Salmon 1984). However, sceptics consider these assays inadequate since predictive accuracy for drug sensitivities range from as low as 20% up to only 67% (reviewed by Kern and Bertelsen 1984). It is, however, important to remember that most of the tumor samples being assayed under these experimental conditions are obtained from the clinically detectable tumors and are in general from heavily pretreated patients. Therefore the bulk of these tumors by clinical experience are likely to be drug resistant. Balance evaluation of the predictive accuracy of these in vitro drug-sensitivity tests must await results from assays carried out on a population of "drug-sensitive" tumors or at least on samples from tumors from untreated patients.

Optimal adjuvant chemotherapy must result in the eradication of the tumor stem cell population. However, stem cells are critical elements in the repopulation, not only of the tumor, but also of normal tissues. Therefore optimal adjuvant chemotherapy must selectively destroy malignant stem cells.

Selective Toxicity on Antitumor Drugs for Malignant Stem Cells: Experimental Evidence. One of the first demonstrations of kinetic differences between normal and malignant stem cells came from experimental laboratory studies by Bruce and his colleagues in 1966. Furthermore they were able to show how these differences might be exploited to achieve increased selective toxicity of antitumor drugs against malignant stem cells. They treated lymphoma-bearing mice with a range of antitumor drugs over a 24-h period and measured

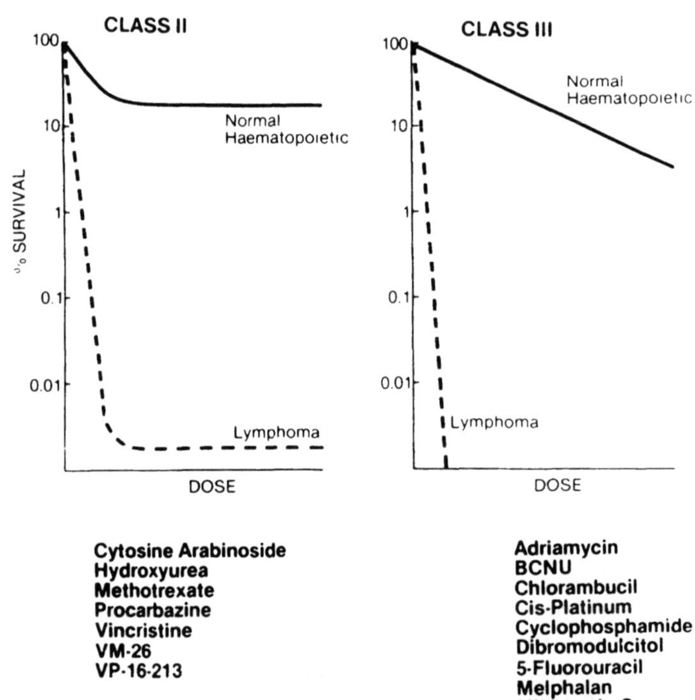

Fig. 6. Kinetic classification of antitumor drugs based on the survival of normal hematopoietic and lymphoma colony-forming cells from mice treated with drugs over 24 h. Treatment in this way resulted in a much greater kill of malignant as opposed to normal stem cells. (Bruce et al. 1966)

the cytotoxic effects on the normal bone marrow stem cells and lymphoma stem cells using the quantitative spleen colony-forming assay. They showed that the drugs tested, when administered over 24 h, fell into two main classes according to the shape of the survival curves obtained: those which did not increase normal bone marrow stem cell kill irrespective of dose (class II) and those where the normal bone marrow stem cell kill did increase with increasing dose (class III). In both classes, however, there was marked slectivity against the lymphoma stem cells, by as much as 10000 times (see Fig. 6). These studies formed the basis for a Kinetic Classification of antitumor drugs. Examples of drugs in these two classes are shown in Fig. 6 and other investigators have extended these studies to include other agents, as reviewed earlier (Hill 1978b, 1982).

This selectivity of both class II and class III drugs against the malignant stem cells appeared to be associated with the fact that in untreated animals most of the normal bone marrow stem cells were resting, while nearly all of the detectable malignant stem cells appeared to be proliferating (Bruce and Valeriote 1968). Therefore, short courses (i.e., over 24 h) of class II and class III drugs, which preferentially kill proliferating cells, would cause much greater kill of malignant as opposed to normal stem cells. If the time of exposure is prolonged, this selectivity is abolished and increasing damage to normal bone marrow occurs (Valeriote and Bruce 1967; Bruce and Meeker 1967). Similarly, if mice were treated after previous injury to the marrow, when hematopoietic stem cells were being recruited to a proliferating state to replace damaged cells, the selectivity of these drugs against malignant stem cells was lost, i.e., the kinetically exploitable difference between normal and malignant stem cells applies for only a limited exposure time of approximately 24-36 h.

A major implication of these studies is that they provided a basis for safer cancer chemotherapy with minimal toxicity to normal bone marrow without compromising antitumor effectiveness. Price and Hill therefore have made a number of predictions, based on these experimental studies, of potential clinical relevance (Price 1973, Hill 1978b; Price and Hill 1981b, 1983), which can be summarized as follows:

1. Bone marrow toxicity will be less if drugs are administered over approximately 24 h in patients.
2. A knowledge of the Kinetic Classification of antitumor drugs is important if chemotherapy is to be administered safely.
3. Toxicity of class II agents to normal stem cells (e.g., in bone marrow) is not dose dependent. Class II drugs therefore may be added to combinations in full dosage, provided the total treatment time does not exceed 36 h.
4. Class III agents in combination will be additively toxic to the marrow, so doses should be reduced proportionately.
5. The practice of giving small daily doses of drugs from either class should be avoided, since normal bone marrow stem cells will be drawn into cycle and killed. This would increase toxicity to normal bone marrow and may reduce the number of malignant stem cells killed because treatment has to be postponed or interrupted.

Clinical Evidence. The first clinical validation of these predictions came from a study showing that bone marrow toxicity from combination chemotherapy using cyclophosphamide, methotrexate, vincristine and 5-fluorouracil in treating miscellaneous "solid" tumors could be significantly reduced if drugs were given over 24 h only (Price and Goldie 1971). It was later shown that Adriamycin could be added to this protocol (see Fig. 7), provided that the doses of the other two class III agents, 5-fluorouracil and cyclophosphamide, were reduced appropriately, without increasing the toxic side effects. This schedule

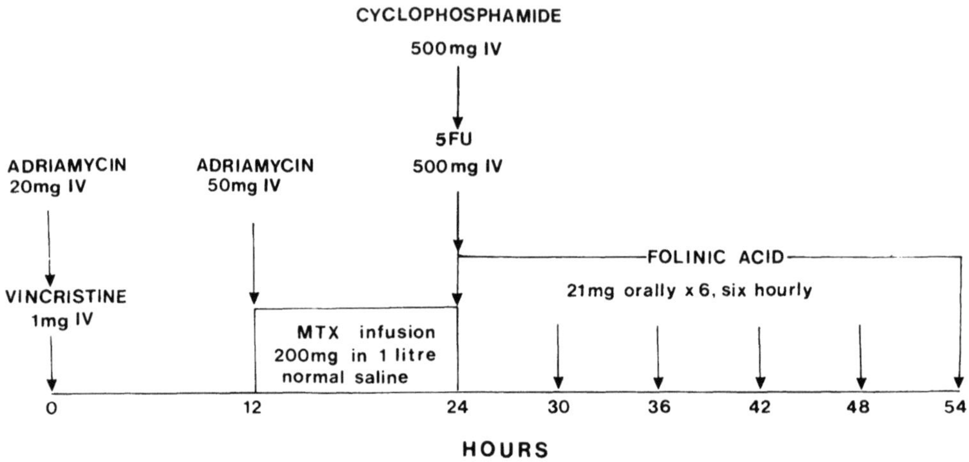

Fig. 7. Kinetically based chemotherapy schedule for breast and uterus (repeat every four weeks)

has been used to treat advanced cancer of the breast or uterus. Subsequently, it has been established that scheduling drugs according to these principles reduces the toxicity but not the effectiveness of combination chemotherapy used in the treatment of a number of advanced cancers including testicular teratomas, lung cancers, ovarian carcinomas, and lymphomas (reviewed recently by Price and Hill 1983). Improved results with markedly reduced toxicity have also been achieved, applying these principles with a four-drug combination in head and neck cancer (Price and Hill 1982; Hill et al. 1984a), as discussed in this volume by Price and Hill.

The prediction that toxicity of class II agents to normal tissues is related more to duration of exposure than to dose was confirmed in 1969 by the demonstration that up to 20000 mg methotrexate (a class I drug) could be given safely over 24 h, while usual doses of 5-100 mg could produce profound marrow depression if given in divided doses over 5 days (Goldie et al. 1972). This study also showed that the value of "high-dose" methotrexate infusions in overcoming drug resistance was remarkably short lived. Current studies have demonstrated that very high doses of other class II agents, such as hydroxyurea or etoposide (VP-16-213), can also be given safely provided that the duration of treatment does not exceed 24 h (Hill and Price 1982; Price and Hill 1983). It remains to be proven whether such usage will translate into improved response rates and so reflect the enhanced tumor cell kill demonstrated with increased duration of drug exposure in our experimental studies, discussed earlier.

The application of these principles has enabled combination chemotherapy to be given more safely clinically than in the past, provided standard medical precautions are always observed (Price and Hill 1981b, 1982). The impact of these kinetically designed protocols on survival is now being investigated. We have, however, already demonstrated that intensive drug combinations can be given safely (Price et al. 1981; Price and Hill 1983), at frequent intervals, especially for the first four or five treatment cycles, since there is no severe myelosuppression, and where tested as initial treatment these chemotherapy protocols do not compromise subsequent surgery or radiotherapy (Price and Hill 1982, also in this volume).

Overall Conclusions

This presentation has highlighted the fact that there is now firm evidence from reliable, reproducible, and carefully controlled experimental and theoretical studies which has permitted the definition of a number of criteria which must be met if optimal adjuvant chemotherapy, aimed at increasing survival, is to be administered. These criteria are:

1. Full-dose, intensive combination chemotherapy should be administered.
2. Intervals between courses of chemotherapy should be kept to a minimum, consistent with clinical tolerance.
3. Initial chemotherapy should integrate successfully and safely with subsequent surgery and/or radiotherapy.

Clinical studies, using the 24-h approach, have shown that these necessary requirements can be met safely. Randomized, prospective, controlled clinical trials should now be carried out to establish whether these necessary requirements are sufficient to improve the cure rates in certain "solid" tumors. In this way the problem of drug resistance may be overcome or circumvented.

Acknowledgements. I am extremely grateful to my colleagues Drs. L. A. Price, L. M. Franks, and J. R. W. Masters for their helpful advice and criticism in the preparation of this presentation. The valuable assistance of Alison Barrow in the typing of the manuscript has been much appreciated.

References

Bruce WR, Meeker BE (1967) Comparison of the sensitivity of hematopoietic colony-forming cells in different proliferative states of 5-fluorouracil. J Natl Cancer Inst 38: 401-405

Bruce WR, Valeriote FA (1968) Normal and malignant stem cells and chemotherapy. In: Proliferation and spread of neoplastic cells. 21st Annual symposium on fundamental cancer research at M. D. Anderson Hospital and Tumor Institute at Houston, Texas. Williams and Wilkins, Baltimore, pp 409-430

Bruce WR, Meeker BE, Valeriote FA (1966) Comparison of the sensitivity of normal hematopoietic and transplanted lymphoma colony-forming cells to chemotherapeutic agents administered in vivo. J Natl Cancer Inst 37: 233-245

Buick RN (1984) Cell heterogeneity in human ovarian carcinoma. J Cell Physiol [Suppl] 3: 117-122

Carnie AB, Lala PK, Osmond DG (1976) Stem cells of renewing cell populations, 1st edn. Academic, New York

DeVita VT (1983) The relationship between tumor mass and resistance to chemotherapy. Cancer 51: 1209-1220

Goldie JH, Coldman AJ (1979) A mathematical model for relating the drug sensitivity of tumors to their spontaneous mutation rate. Cancer Treat Rep 63: 1727-1733

Goldie JH, Price LA, Harrap KR (1972) Methotrexate toxicity: correlation with duration of administration, plasma levels, dose and excretion pattern. Eur J Cancer 8: 409-414

Goldie JH, Coldman AJ, Gudauskas GA (1982) Rationale for the use of alternating non-cross-resistant chemotherapy. Cancer Treat Rep 66: 439-449

Hamburger AW, Salmon SE (1977) Primary bio-assay of human tumor stem cells. Science 197: 461-463

Hill BT (1978 a) The management of human "solid" tumors: some observations on the irrelevance of traditional cell cycle kinetics and the value of certain recent concepts. Cell Biol Int Rep 2: 215-230

Hill BT (1978 b) Cancer chemotherapy - the relevance of certain concepts of cell cycle kinetics. Biochem Biophys Acta 516: 389-417

Hill BT (1983) Biochemical and cell kinetic aspects of drug resistance. In: Bruchovsky N, Goldie JH (eds) Drug and hormone resistance in neoplasia, vol I. Basic concepts. CRC Press, Boca Raton, pp 21-53

Hill BT (1983) An overview of clonogenic assays for human tumor biopsies. In: Dendy PP, Hill BT (eds) Human tumor drug sensitivity testing *in vitro*. Academic, London, pp 91-102

Hill BT, Baserga R (1975) The cell cycle and its significance for cancer treatment. Cancer Treat Rev 2: 159-175

Hill BT, Bellamy AS (1984) Establishment of an etoposide-resistant human epithelial tumor cell line in vitro: characterization of patterns of cross-resistance and drug sensitivities. Int J Cancer 33: 599-608

Hill BT, Price LA (1982) An experimental biological basis for increasing the therapeutic index of clinical cancer therapy. Ann NY Acad Sci 397: 72-87

Hill BT, Price LA, Busby E, MacRae K, Shaw JH (1984a) Positive impact of initial 24-hour combination chemotherapy without cis-platinum on 6-year survival figures in advanced squamous cell carcinomas of the head and neck. In: Jones SE, Salmon E (eds) Adjuvant therapy of cancer IV. Grune and Stratton, Orlando, pp 97-106

Hill BT, Shaw JH, Dalley VM, Price LA (1984b) 24-hour combination chemotherapy without cisplatin in patients with recurrent or metastatic head and neck cancer. Am J Clin Oncol 7: 335-340

Hill BT, Whelan RDH, Bellamy AS (1984c) Fractionated radiation exposure in vitro results in altered drug responses in murine and human continuous tumor cell lines. Proc Am Assoc Cancer Res 25: 331

Hill BT, Whelan RDH, Hosking LK, Ward BG, Gibby EM (1984d) The value of human tumor continuous cell lines for investigating aspects of the methodologies used for in vitro drug sensitivity testing. In: Salmon SE, Trent JM (eds) Human tumor cloning. Grune and Stratton, Orlando, pp 487-496

Hill BT, Whelan RDH, Bellamy AS, Rupniak HT (1985) Pitfalls in the soft agar clonogenic assays: recommendations for improving colony-forming effiencies and the potential value of cell lines derived from head and neck tumors. In: Chretien P (ed) Head and neck cancer. Decker, Philadelphia (in press)

Holland JK, Glidewell O, Cooper RG (1980) Adverse effect of radiotherapy on adjuvant chemotherapy of breast cancer. Surg Gynecol Obstet 150: 817-821

Kern DH, Bertelsen CA (1984) Present status of chemosensitivity assays. Int Adv Surg Oncol 7: 187-213

Mann BD, Kern DH, Giuliano AE, Burk MW, Campbell MA, Kaiser LR, Morton DL (1982) Clinical correlations with drug sensitivities in the clonogenic assay. Arch Surg 117: 33-36

McCullough EA, Till JE (1971) Regulatory mechanisms acting on hematopoietic stem cells: some clinical implications. Am J Pathol 65: 601-619

Paulson DF, Einhorn L, Peckham M, Williams SD (1982) Cancer of the testis. In: DeVita VT, Hellman S, Rosenberg SA (eds) Cancer: principles and practice of oncology. Lippincott, Philadelphia, pp 786-822

Price LA (1973) The application of a kinetic model to the clinical use of antitumor drugs. In: Shedden WIH (ed) Proceedings of the 3rd Eli Lilly symposium on the vinca alkaloids in the chemotherapy of malignant disease. Sherraff, Cheshire, pp 35-40

Price LA, Goldie JH (1971) Multiple drug therapy for disseminated malignant disease. Br Med J 4: 336-339

Price LA, Hill BT (1981a). Safe and effective combination chemotherapy without cis-platinum for squamous cell carcinomas of the head and neck. Cancer Treat Rep 65: (Suppl 1) 149-154

Price LA, Hill BT (1981b) Safer chemotherapy using a kinetically-based approach: clinical applications. In: Price LA, Hill BT, Ghilchik M (eds) Safer cancer chemotherapy. Bailliere Tindall, London, pp 9-18

Price LA, Hill BT (1982) Safe and effective induction chemotherapy without cisplatin for squamous cell carcinoma of the head and neck: impact on complete response rate and survival at five years, following local therapy. Med Ped Oncol 10: 535-548

Price LA, Hill BT (1983) An experimentally-based safe method of administering intensive cancer chemotherapy: prospects for increased survival in patients with 'solid' tumors in the next decade. S Afr Med J 64: 987-994

Price LA, Hill BT, Ghilchik M (1981) Safer cancer chemotherapy. Bailliere Tindall, London

Rupniak HT, Whelan RD, Hill BT (1983) Concentration and time- dependent inter-relationships for antitumor drug cytotoxicities against tumor cells in vitro. Int J Cancer 32: 7-12

Salmon SE (1984) Preclinical and clinical applications of chemosensitivity testing with a human tumor colony assay. In: Salmon SE, Trent JM (eds) Human tumor cloning. Grune and Stratton, Orlando, pp 499-508

Schabel FM (1977) Surgical adjuvant chemotherapy of metastatic murine tumors. Cancer 40: 558-568

Shackney SE, McCormack GW, Cuchural GJ (1978) Growth rate patterns of solid tumors and their relation to responsiveness to therapy. Ann Intern Med 89: 107-121

Skipper HE, Schabel FM, Wilcox WS (1965) Experimental evaluation of potential anticancer drugs. XIV. Further study of certain basic concepts underlying chemotherapy of leukemia. Cancer Chemother Rep 45: 5-28

Steel GC (1977) Growth kinetics of tumors, 1st edn. Clarendon, Oxford, pp 1-351

Thomson SP, Moon TE, Meyskens FL (1984) Kinetics of clonogenic melanoma cell proliferation and the limits of growth within a bilayer agar system. J Cell Physiol 121: 114-124

Valeriote FA, Bruce WR (1967) Comparison of the sensitivity of hematopoietic colony-forming cells in different proliferative states to vinblastine. J Natl Cancer Inst 38: 393-399

Valeriote FA, van Putten LM (1975) Proliferation-dependent cytotoxicity of anticancer agents: a review. Cancer Res 35: 2619-2630

Von Hoff DD, Casper J, Bradley E, Sandbank J, Jones D, Makuch R (1981) Association between human tumor colony forming assay results and response of an individual patient's tumor to chemotherapy. Am J Med 70: 1027-1032

Wilcox WS, Griswold DP, Laster WR, Schabel SM, Skipper HE (1965) Experimental evaluation of potential anticancer agents. XVII. Kinetics of growth and regression after treatment of certain solid tumors. Cancer Chemother Rep 47: 27-39

Wolf GT, Chretien PB (1981) The chemotherapy and immunotherapy of head and neck cancer. In: Suen JY, Myers EN (eds) Cancer of the head and neck. Churchill Livingstone, New York, pp 782-820

Young RC, Knapp RC, Perez CA (1982) Cancer of the ovary. In: DeVita VT, Hellman S, Rosenberg SA (eds) Cancer: principles and practice of oncology. Lippincott, Philadelphia, pp 884-913

Adjuvant Therapy for Breast Cancer: A Brief Overview of the NSABP Experience and Some Thoughts on Neoadjuvant Chemotherapy

B. Fisher

University of Pittsburgh, Medical School, 3550 Terrace Street, Pittsburgh, PA 15261, USA

Introduction

When the first trials evaluating postoperative adjuvant therapy for the treatment of primary breast cancer were being designed in the early 1970s, it was considered a prerequisite that the drugs employed be those which proved to be of benefit in patients with advanced disease. Similarly, when embarking upon trials to evaluate the concept of neoadjuvant therapy (preoperative) it seems entirely appropriate that the therapies considered for use be those which have demonstrated an advantage when used postoperatively. In fact, the question still remains in the minds of many as to whether postoperative adjuvant chemotherapy has resulted in a benefit and, if so, in what patients. Of course, there remains the possibility, but unlikely, that nonadvantageous postoperative therapies might be beneficial in the neoadjuvant setting. Nonetheless, logic would dictate that as a starting point regimens of proven worth be employed.

The purpose of this presentation is to present a brief overview of some of the findings obtained in the National Surgical Adjuvant Breast and Bowel Project (NSABP) trials employing postoperative adjuvant chemotherapy, and some laboratory information as well as some personal comments about the use of neoadjuvant therapy. It is my opinion that the term "neoadjuvant" therapy is a neologism which is a poor and inappropriate one which should be abandoned before it becomes more firmly fixed in its use. Since "neo-" is a prefix meaning "new," it fails to connote that which it is intended to portray, i.e., preoperative therapy. Moreover, a therapy which is considered for the moment to be new may rapidly lose that characterization but its appellation will persist.

NSABP trials of postoperative adjuvant therapy

The current series of NSABP protocols was introduced in 1972 with the specific aim of determining the propriety of adjuvant chemotherapy in patients with primary operable stage II breast cancer. Consonant with this effort was the commitment not merely to compare various therapeutic regimens but to enhance the biological understanding of breast cancer. Since 1972, six randomized prospective clinical trials have been completed accruing over 5500 patients. The studies were carried out sequentially, and the underlying biological theme of each study was in part influenced by the results obtained from the previous protocol. A spectrum of therapeutic interventions was evolved ranging from the simplest of single-agent chemotherapy to more complex multiple-drug regimens. The initial studies were viewed as therapeutic probes and were aimed at identifying those patient subsets likely to respond to one, two, or three chemotherapeutic agents. As early as 1972, it

Recent Results in Cancer Research. Vol 103

Table 1. NSABP adjuvant chemotherapy trials positive-node patients

Protocol	Regimen	Interval	Accrual
B-05	Placebo vs. P	9/72-2/75	370
B-07	P vs. PF	2/75-2/76	741
B-09	PF vs. PFT	1/77-4/80	1891
B-08	PF vs. PMF	4/76-4/77	737
B-11	PF vs. PAF	6/81-9/84	707
B-12	PFT vs. PAFT	6/81-9/84	1025

P, L-phenylalanine mustard; *F*, 5-fluorouracil; *T*, tamoxifen; *M*, methotrexate; *A*, adriamycin

was appreciated that single-agent chemotherapy in the form of L-phenylalanine mustard (L-PAM) was unlikely to represent the most effective regimen in the adjuvant setting since it had previously been demonstrated that combination chemotherapy was superior to L-PAM in metastatic disease (Greenspan 1966; Cooper 1969). Despite this observation, the decision was made to proceed with a study comparing L-PAM to placebo with the expressed intent of providing a frame of reference for the evaluation of more complex therapeutic options. Moreover, there was evidence from experimental models to suggest that single agents might be highly efficacious in the adjuvant setting. The expectations from the L-PAM study were modest and it was anticipated that superior results would be forthcoming from subsequent protocols. It was hypothesized in keeping with the burgeoning knowledge related to tumor heterogeneity that these studies would be successful in characterizing discrete patient subsets that were likely to respond to the various therapeutic interventions.

Protocol B-05, a double-blind study comparing L-PAM with placebo, was started in September 1972 and terminated in February 1975 after 370 patients with histologically positive nodes were entered (Table 1). L-PAM was given on 5 successive days of a 6-week cycle. This study as well as the five subsequent NSABP adjuvant therapy protocols for stage II disease mandated that therapy be administered for a duration of 2 years. Following the demonstration of an early benefit from single-agent L-PAM and in keeping with the overall stepwise strategy, protocol B-07 was introduced in order to ascertain the utility of adding 5-FU to L-PAM. The design of protocol B-07 was similar to that of B-05 and consisted of a two-arm protocol in which single-agent L-PAM was compared with the two-drug combination of L-PAM and 5-FU (PF). Between February 1975 and May 1976, 741 patients were randomized. The third trial in the series, protocol B-08, compared the two-drug combination PF, as administered in protocol B-07, with the three-drug combination in which methotrexate was added to the PF regimen (PMF). Between April 1976 and April 1977, 737 patients were randomized into this study. Following results indicating that the addition of methotrexate failed to enhance the effect of PF, three additional studies were instituted. One, protocol B-09, accrued 1891 patients between January 1977 and May 1980. Women were randomized to receive adjuvant chemotherapy consisting of L-phenylalanine mustard and 5-FU (PF) with and without tamoxifen. The chemotherapeutic agents employed as well as the decision not to utilize tamoxifen without chemotherapy was directly based on the results of the three previous NSABP chemotherapy trials. Since it had been demonstrated that PF could alter the natural history of breast cancer in more patient subsets than P, the PF combination provided a logical baseline for assessing the effect of tamoxifen.

Between June 1981 and September 1984, 1732 patients were entered into protocols B-11 and B-12. These studies were designed to determine whether adding Adriamycin to PF would result in an incremental benefit in a setting where the addition of methotrexate had been without value. The six NSABP sequential protocols have all completed patient accrual. They represent the largest available clinical trial experience with adjuvant chemotherapy in the stage II setting.

Results

Protocol B-05: Placebo versus L-PAM. An update of the results of protocol B-05 indicates that there continues to be a prolongation in disease-free survival for patients treated with L-PAM compared with those receiving placebo after 10 years average time on study, corroborating the conclusions of previous reports (Fisher et al. 1975, 1977, 1980). Examination of all patients, without regard for age and nodal status, indicates that there was an overall significant advantage with respect to disease-free survival for those women receiving L-PAM ($P=0.07$). Age appears to be an important discriminant in characterizing the benefit of L-PAM. The effect of L-PAM on disease-free survival was not uniform and selectively benefited those ≦49 years ($P=0.03$, Fig. 1). Further analysis of patients ≦ 49 years of age according to the number of histologically positive nodes once again discloses a nonuniform response to therapy. Patients ≦49 years of age who are characterized by one to three positive nodes sustained the greatest response whereas the patient cohort with ≧ four positive nodes appeared to be more resistant (Fig. 2). Patients ≧ 50 years continue to demonstrate no benefit from single-agent L-PAM and the disease-free survival benefit noted in patients ≦49 with one to three positive nodes has been translated into a significant difference in survival (Fig. 3).

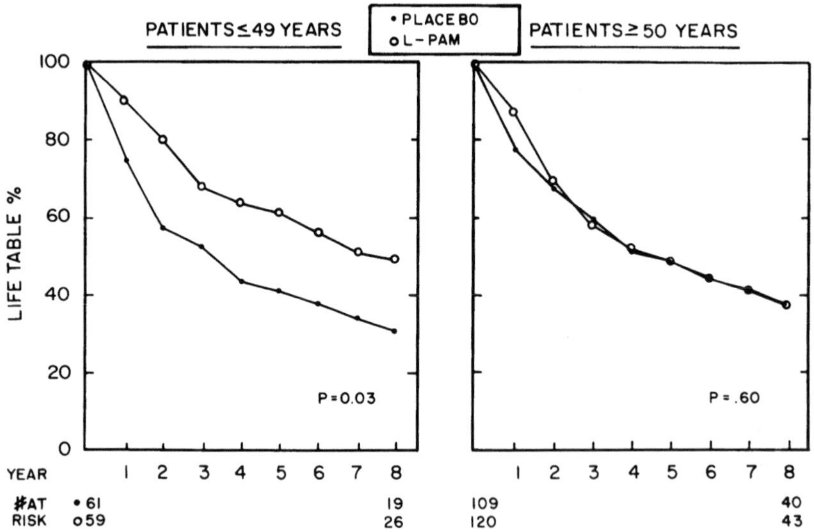

Fig. 1. Placebo vs. L-PAM disease-free survival according to age

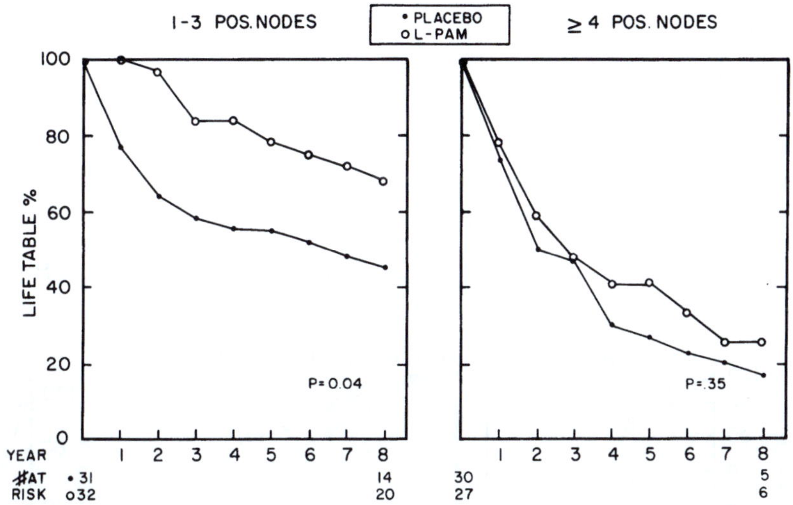

Fig. 2. Placebo vs. L-PAM disease-free survival: patients ≦49 years of age according to nodes

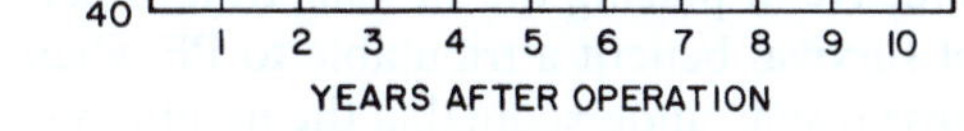

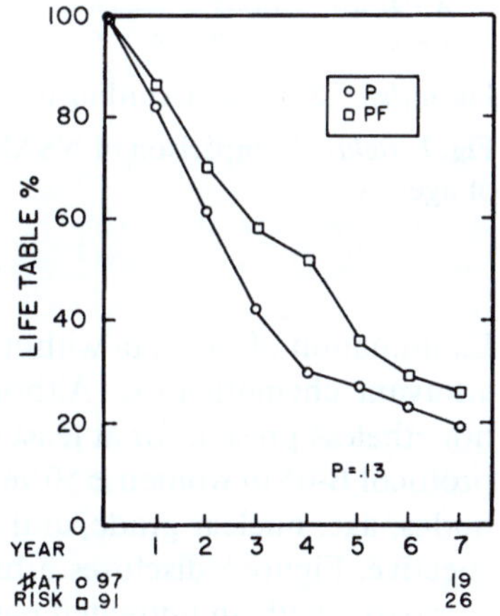

Fig. 3 *(left).* Survival: patients ≦49 years of age with one to three positive nodes

Fig. 4 *(right).* P vs. PF disease-free survival: patients ≧50 years of age with ≧four positive nodes

Protocol B-07: P versus PF. The propriety of adding 5-FU to L-PAM was addressed in protocol B-07. In contrast to the benefit achieved by L-PAM when used as a single agent, the addition of 5-FU to L-PAM improved the disease-free survival in patients ≧ 50 years over and above that achieved by single-agent L-PAM. Further analyzing the group of women ≧ 50 years according to the number of histologically positive axillary nodes disclosed that the PF advantage was apparent predominantly in women with ≧ four positive nodes (Fig. 4). This advantage was in evidence for both disease-free survival and survival for up to 6 years following the commencement of the study. Beyond the 6-year interval the differences attributable to the addition of 5-FU to L-PAM in patients ≧ 50 years with four or more positive nodes have become attenuated and are no longer statistically significant.

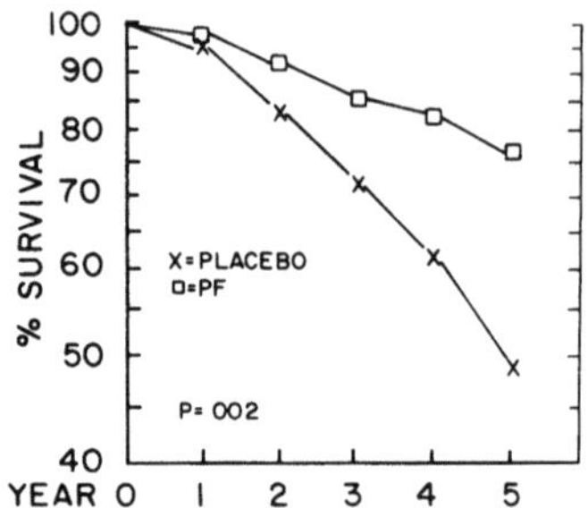

Fig. 5. Survival with PF vs. placebo: ≧50 years of age

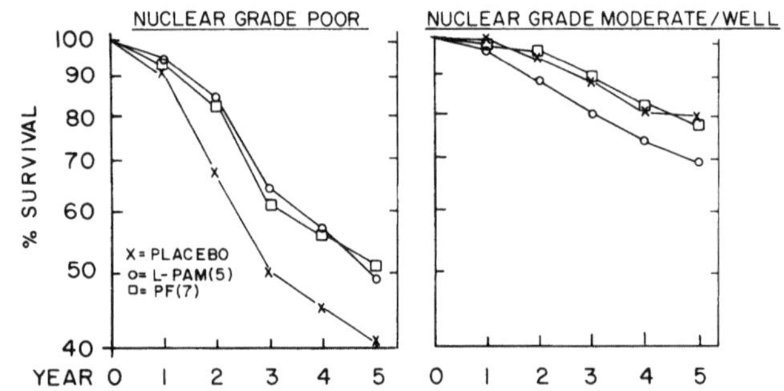

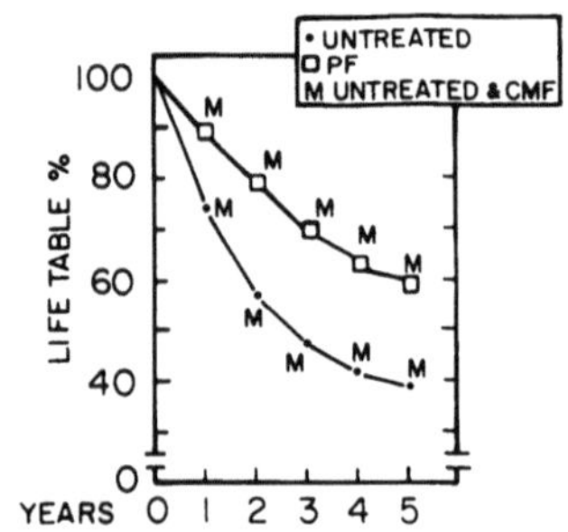

Fig. 6 *(left).* Survival according to nuclear grade

Fig. 7 *(right).* Comparison of NSABP PF with Milan CMF: disease-free survival patients ≦49 years of age

Examination of the data within each protocol belies the incremental gains made utilizing adjuvant chemotherapy. Although the benefit obtained with PF was transient, it was nonetheless present for at least 6 years. Comparison of the PF results with the placebo of protocol B-05 in women ≧ 50 years and adjusting for imbalances in the number of positive nodes, age, nuclear grade, and tumor size is effective in placing the PF benefit into perspective. Figure 5 discloses a highly significant survival benefit attributable to PF when compared with an untreated patient cohort. These results underscore that the natural history of breast cancer in women ≧ 50 years has been favorably altered. Moreover, the use of the traditional subset characteristics based on age and the number of positive nodes may overlook an important interaction associated with another discriminant. Preliminary analyses of the data from protocols B-05 and B-07 indicate that nuclear grade may be an important indicator of chemotherapy responsiveness. When survival was related to nuclear grade for P and PF an impressive benefit was apparent for nuclear-grade poor tumors but not for well-differentiated lesions (Fig. 6).

It is of interest to obtain a comparative overview of the magnitude of the differences obtained by PF and those achieved with CMF. In order that this comparison may be addressed, the cumulative PF data from NSABP protocols B-05, B-07, and B-08 were combined and compared with the pooled NSABP data for untreated patients in protocol B-05 and the radical mastectomy group in protocol B-04 (Fig. 7). The results obtained with CMF from the Milan data (Bonadonna and Valagussa 1982) have been superimposed on the PF life table graphs. When the data were examined in this manner for premenopausal women or those ≦ 49 years (the group demonstrating the greatest responsiveness), the

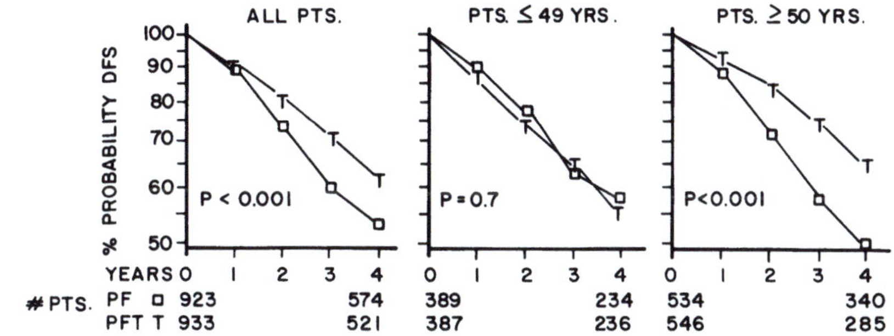

Fig. 8. Disease-free survival (DFS) in all randomized patients regardless of receptor status

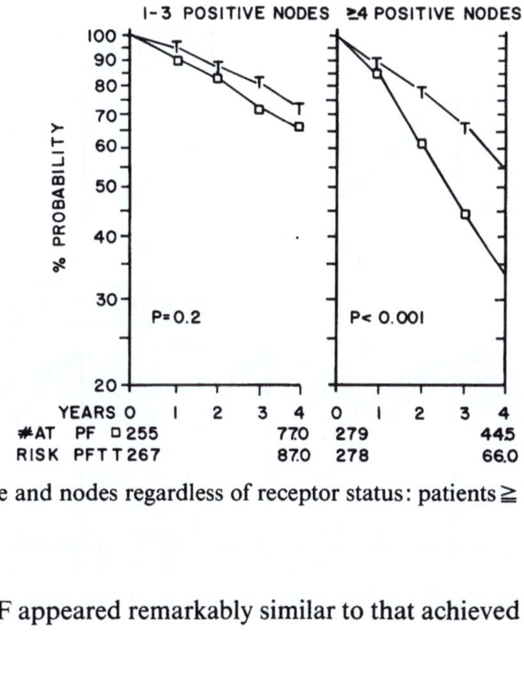

Fig. 9. B-09 disease-free survival relative to age and nodes regardless of receptor status: patients ≧ 50 years of age

magnitude of differences achieved with PF appeared remarkably similar to that achieved with CMF.

Protocol B-08: PF versus PMF. The next sequential protocol in this chemotherapy series addressed the addition of methotrexate to L-PAM and 5-FU (PMF). When all patients were analyzed without regard for age and nodal status, no differences were noted between the PF- and PMF-treated patients for as long as 96 months mean time on study. Further analysis of the data according to age and nodal status consistently failed to demonstrate a benefit for the three-drug combination when contrasted with PF.

Protocol B-09: PF versus PFT. Since the initial aims of this study did not include any restrictions on tumor receptor status, it became mandatory first to analyze the data according to traditional patient subsets without regard for tumor receptor content. Examination of disease-free survival for all patients irrespective of age and the number of positive nodes disclosed a significant prolongation when tamoxifen was added to PF ($P = 0.0001$, Fig. 8). Further analysis according to age demonstrated a disparate response in that patients ≧ 50 years benefited from tamoxifen ($P < 0.001$), whereas women ≦ 49 years appeared to be

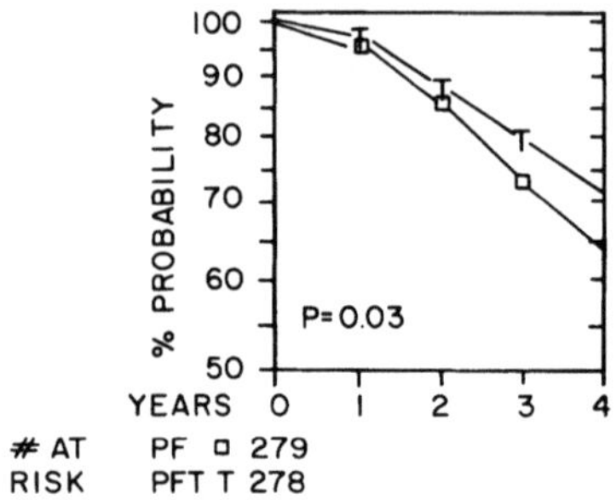

Fig. 10. Survival regardless of receptor status: patients ≧ 50 years of age with ≧ four positive nodes

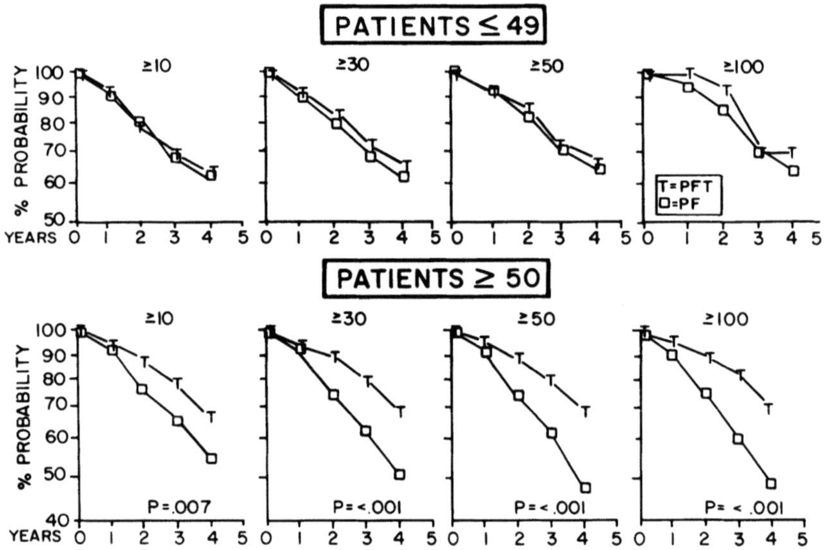

Fig. 11. PF vs. PFT B-09 disease-free survival relative to ER

resistant. Subdivision of the ≧ 50 years cohort according to the number of positive nodes indicated that the largest increment in disease-free survival occurred in the four or more positive node subset ($P > 0.0001$). Thus, the benefit attributed to tamoxifen for all patients without regard for receptor status was derived exclusively from the contribution of women ≧ 50 years of age particularly if they had ≧ four positive nodes (Fig. 9). The disease-free survival benefit noted in women ≧ 50 years of age with ≧ four positive nodes has been translated into a significant prolongation in actual survivorship ($P = 0.03$, Fig. 10).

Examination of disease-free survival according to quantitative tumor estrogen receptor content indicated that no benefit for tamoxifen was observed in patients whose tumor estrogen receptors were < 10 fmol (data not shown). The results were then evaluated according to quantitative tumor estrogen receptor content irrespective of age and nodal status.

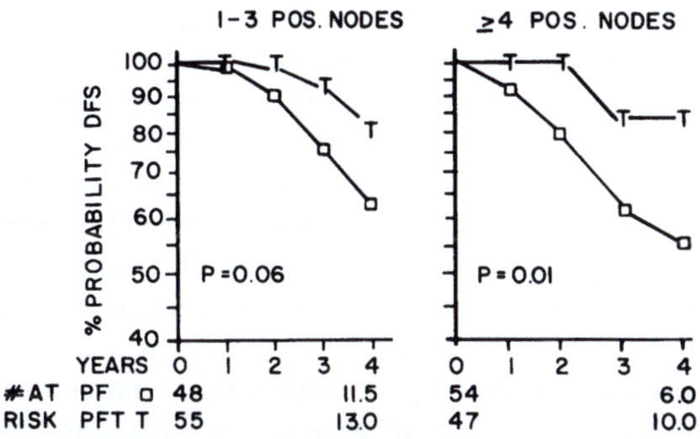

Fig. 12. Disease-free survival in patients ≧ 50 years of age: tumor ER ≧ 50 fmol

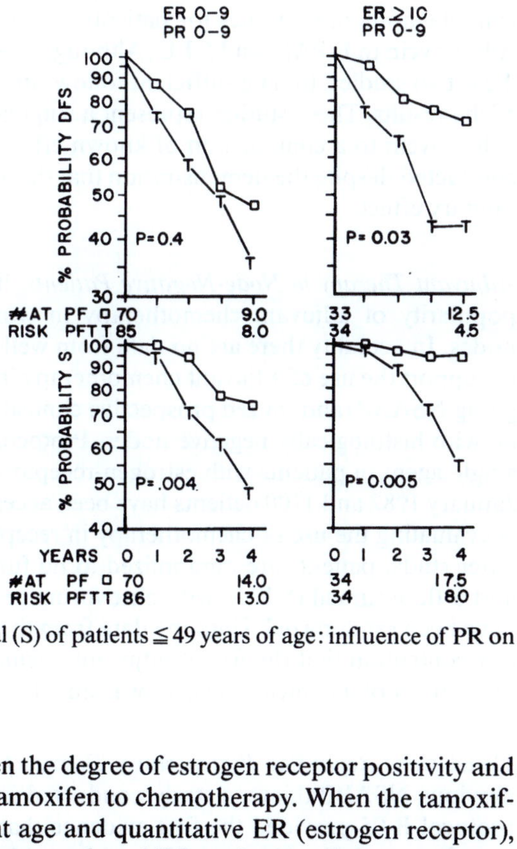

Fig. 13. Disease-free survival (DFS) and survival (S) of patients ≦ 49 years of age: influence of PR on ER

There appeared to be a relationship between the degree of estrogen receptor positivity and the benefit attributable to the addition of tamoxifen to chemotherapy. When the tamoxifen data were analyzed according to patient age and quantitative ER (estrogen receptor), once again, a marked heterogeneous response to the addition of tamoxifen was encountered. Women ≦ 49 years of age failed to benefit from the addition of tamoxifen even if the tumor ER content was ≧ 100 fmol/mg (Fig. 11). It became evident that the prolongation in disease-free survival noted for all receptor-positive patients was derived exclusively from women ≧ 50 years of age where highly significant differences were apparent; these differences have not as yet been translated into a survival advantage. Further examination of the cohort of patients ≧ 50 years of age according to the number of positive nodes indicated that the tamoxifen benefit was present in both the one to three and ≧ four positive node subsets but was more impressive in the latter group (Fig. 12).

This study was also instructive in underscoring the potential dangers of the injudicious application of adjuvant therapy. In contrast to the benefit achieved by tamoxifen, there was also observed an unanticipated negative influence. It was previously pointed out that women ≦ 49 years of age failed to benefit from the addition of tamoxifen to PF chemotherapy regardless of receptor level. If tamoxifen was administered to patients ≦ 49 years of age whose tumor progesterone receptors were < 10 fmol, not only did these patients not benefit from tamoxifen, but there was a significant decrease in disease-free survival and survival when compared with similar patients receiving only PF (Fig. 13). This negative effect did not reduce disease-free survival and survival to levels below those documented in patients not treated with *any* adjuvant therapy, but the addition of tamoxifen to this group appeared to attenuate the beneficial response observed with chemotherapy.

Protocol B-11 and B-12: PF versus PAF. The final protocols in this stepwise series of adjuvant chemotherapy studies for patients with positive nodes address the utility of adding Adriamycin to L-PAM and 5-FU. Although over 1700 patients have been randomized into these two studies, to date sufficient follow-up is unavailable to allow meaningful analysis of the results. These studies represent a singular endeavor in which the benefit of adding Adriamycin to a combination of known efficacy is being determined. This protocol was conducted despite the demonstration that the addition of methotrexate to PF was without salutary effect.

Adjuvant Therapy in Node-Negative Patients. It is disconcerting to witness the increasing popularity of adjuvant chemotherapy in women with histologically negative axillary nodes. In actuality there are no data from well-controlled studies that are as yet available to support the use of adjuvant chemotherapy in node-negative patients. There are two ongoing NSABP randomized prospective clinical trials evaluating adjuvant therapy in women with histologically negative nodes. Protocol B-14 addresses the use of tamoxifen as a single agent in patients with estrogen-receptor-positive tumors. This study was started in January 1982 and 1100 patients have been accessed to date. The companion protocol B-13 is evaluating the use of chemotherapy in receptor-negative node-negative patients. In the latter study, patients are randomized to no further treatment or sequential methotrexate and 5-fluorouracil (5-FU), with citrovorum rescue. Since August 1981, over 300 patients have been randomized. Until the data from these and other studies become available, it is our contention that the use of adjuvant chemotherapy in node-negative women outside the context of a clinical trial is unwarranted.

Conclusions Regarding Postoperative Therapy from NSABP Trials. With the exception of a previous NSABP thiotepa study conducted in 1958 (Fisher et al. 1968), the findings of protocol B-05 provided the first evidence that adjuvant chemotherapy can prolong disease-free survival and survival in patients with positive nodes. These results are therefore noteworthy for their conceptual contribution rather than the limited therapeutic efficacy attributable to single-agent L-PAM. The demonstration that the effect of L-PAM was not uniform and selectively benefited those patients who are ≦ 49 years of age underscores the heterogeneous response to adjuvant therapy. The findings that patients ≦ 49 years of age with one to three positive nodes sustained the greatest benefit further emphasizes the lack of uniform response to therapy. As a consequence of this demonstration, the examination of adjuvant therapy response only in terms of *all* patients without regard for age and nodal status is anachronistic and disregards the behavior of the disease.

The heterogeneous response to therapy is in further evidence when patients receiving PF are compared with those treated with L-PAM alone. The addition of 5-FU to L-PAM resulted in a transient increment in disease-free survival and survival over the use of L-PAM which was most evident for patients ≧ 50 years of age. An appreciation for the efficacy of the PF regimen may be obtained by contrasting disease-free survival in PF-treated patients with those patients untreated with chemotherapy. Even in patients ≧ 50 years of age a significant advantage in survival was observed. An enhanced understanding of chemotherapy responsiveness has resulted from the observation that poor nuclear grade tumors may be more responsive to adjuvant therapy, thus providing a new and potentially powerful discriminant for predicting the outcome of chemotherapy intervention. The failure of the three-drug combination PMF to achieve a benefit over and above that observed with PF for any of the patient subsets challenges the tenet that combinations containing a greater number of agents are more effective in the adjuvant setting.

The protocols in this series, assessing the propriety of adding Adriamycin to L-PAM and 5-FU, constitute the definitive test of whether adding further agents to the PF combination will result in an enhanced disease-free survival and survival. If the addition of that agent is unable to increase the efficacy of that combination, a serious reassessment of the current multiple-agent approach would have to be considered.

The results indicate that the addition of tamoxifen to PF can prolong disease-free survival over and above that noted with PF alone. The response to tamoxifen was not uniform and the benefit observed when all patients were evaluated was contributed exclusively by women ≧ 50 years of age and was associated with tumor ER and PR (progesterone receptor) content. In this latter group (≧ 50 years of age), as the tumor quantitative ER level increased there appeared to be a corresponding decrease in the incidence of treatment failure. This was true in both the one to three and ≧ four positive-node categories. When the data were examined without regard for tumor receptor status, the disease-free survival advantage attributable to tamoxifen in women ≧ 50 years of age with ≧ four positive nodes was translated into an actual survival benefit.

To place the effect of tamoxifen into perspective, it may be of some value to review the NSABP cumulative observations with the first generation of adjuvant therapy trials (Table 2). If one selects PF as being illustrative of responsiveness to chemotherapy it is evident that those women < 49 years of age demonstrate the greatest sensitivity to adjuvant chemotherapy. Of this group, patients with one to three positive nodes are most responsive. In contrast there was a small benefit noted in women ≧ 50 years of age which was de-

Table 2. NSABP cumulative PF experience

	PF	T
≦ 49 years of age	+ + +	–
One to three nodes	+ + +	–
> Four nodes	–	–
≧ 50 years of age	+	+ + +
One to three nodes	–	+ +
≧ Four nodes	+	+ + +

P, L-phenylalanine mustard; *T*, tamoxifen

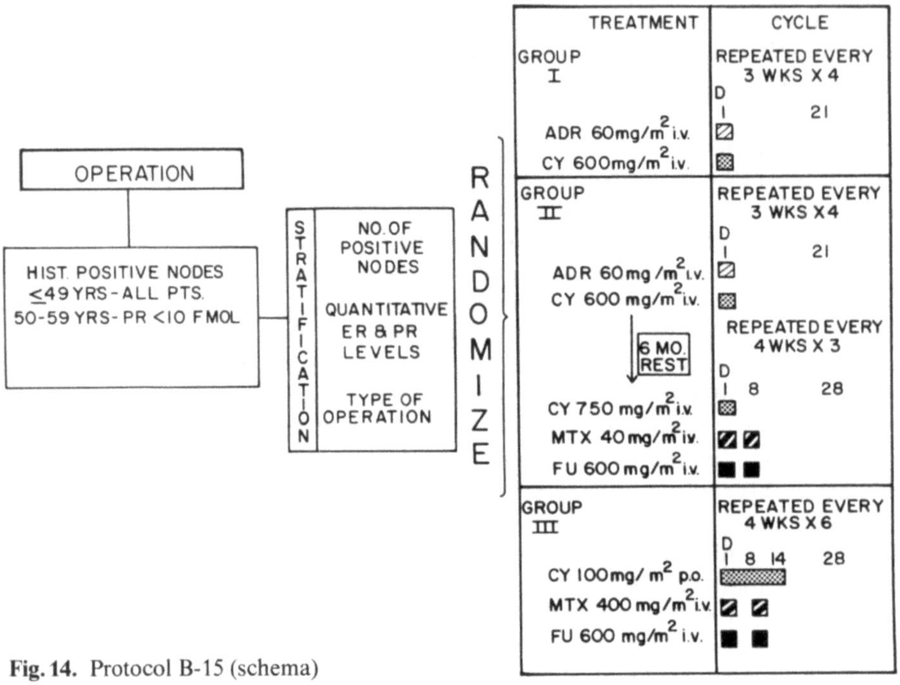

Fig. 14. Protocol B-15 (schema)

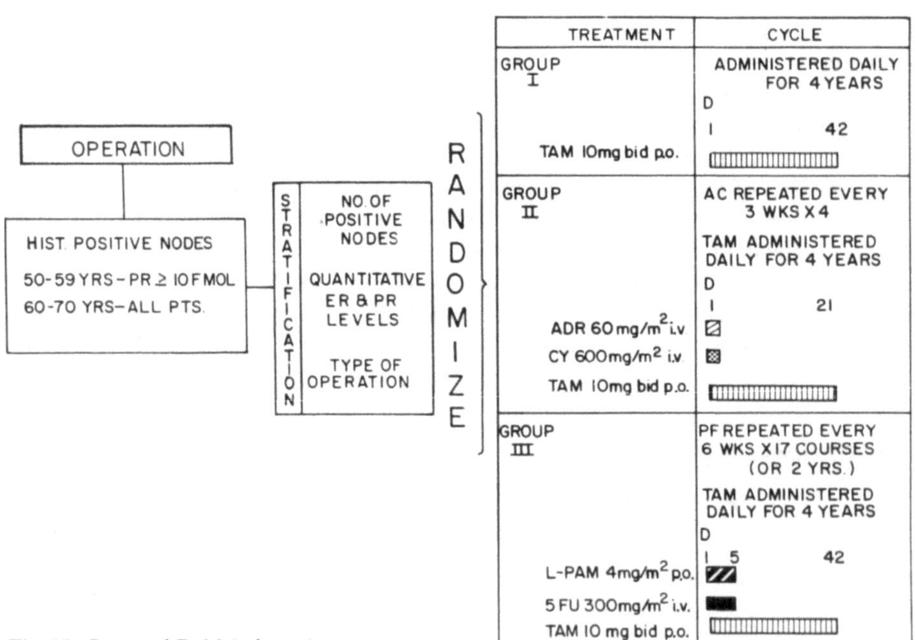

Fig. 15. Protocol B-16 (schema)

rived exclusively from patients with ≧ four positive nodes. The addition of tamoxifen to PF failed to improve on the prolongation in disease-free survival noted in the group most sensitive to chemotherapy, namely, patients ≦ 49 years of age. Contrariwise those women that were relatively resistant to PF, women ≧ 50 years of age, sustained the greatest benefit from the addition of tamoxifen.

The propriety of administering tamoxifen alone or tamoxifen together with chemotherapy is a theme being explored in the current generation of NSABP protocols. A major study in that regard (NSABP protocol B-14) is limited to node-negative receptor-positive patients, randomizes women to tamoxifen or placebo, and has thus far accrued over 1200 patients. The results will no doubt contribute to the elucidation of the role of tamoxifen as a single agent.

In all six NSABP protocols there was a significant advantage in disease-free survival that was apparent within the 1st year of therapy. This effect was uniform in that the benefit was observed regardless of patient age or the number of positive nodes. This observation suggests that the biological perturbations which occur with adjuvant chemotherapy are in evidence as early as the first few cycles of treatment. It was therefore hypothesized that the first few cycles could be exploited for increased gain by utilizing short intensive therapy. The current NSABP protocol B-15 (Fig. 14) in node-positive patients is addressing the utility of a short intensive chemotherapy regimen consisting of Adriamycin and cyclophosphamide (AC). This study is limited to patients who failed to demonstrate a benefit from the addition of tamoxifen to chemotherapy. Whether the potential gains from this initial short and intensive regimen can be improved upon will be ascertained by a reinduction regimen consisting of high-dose parenteral CMF to be introduced 6 months following AC administration.

In women who responded to tamoxifen (women ≧ 50 years of age) the interaction of tamoxifen with chemotherapy is being evaluated in protocol B-16 (Fig. 15). In this study patients are randomized to tamoxifen alone, short intensive AC together with tamoxifen and to the standard PFT regimen. This study will determine whether the PFT effect can be duplicated by the use of tamoxifen alone without chemotherapy or whether the use of tamoxifen with another potentially more effective chemotherapy regimen (AC) will provide further gains.

Perioperative Therapy

Several biological premises provide justification for considering the use of perioperative chemotherapy. One relates to the effect that removal of a primary tumor has on the growth kinetics of metastases. Our studies have demonstrated that with 24 h following removal of primary C3H mammary tumor, there is an increase in the labeling index (LI) of a distant tumor focus that persists for between 7 and 10 days (Gunduz et al. 1979). There is also a decrease in tumor doubling time and a measurable increase in tumor size that become apparent about a week following primary tumor removal. The tumor growth is probably a result of the conversion of noncycling cells in G_0 phase into proliferating cells, cells that should be more vulnerable to cytostatic agents. The rapidity of the onset of the kinetic changes and their relatively short duration provides a suitable rationale for the use of chemotherapy as soon as possible following tumor removal. Investigations carried out by use in an animal model have indeed indicated that chemotherapy had a more favorable effect when given on the day of tumor removal than 3 days later, when the LI of metastases was at a peak, and it was least effective when given at a time when the LI had returned to the preoperative level (Fisher et al. 1983). The greatest benefit occurred when the chemotherapy was given prior to operation. Use at that time completely prevented the increase in LI, more effectively suppressed tumor growth, and prolonged survival to a greater extent than was noted under any other circumstance. This suggests that for more effective control of metastases, chemotherapy had best be employed before or at the time of primary tumor removal.

The mechanism whereby removal of a primary tumor exerts its effect on metastases is worthy of investigation. What mediates such a phenomenon and what characterizes the cells that respond to the stimulus? It hardly needs pointing out that the kinetic changes observed by us and by others (Schiffer et al. 1978; Simpson-Herren et al. 1976) in animal models provide no assurance that a similar phenomenon takes place following the removal in the human of all or even some primary tumor of the same or different types. Moreover, there is no assurance that the temporal pattern of the kinetic changes in the animal and in the patient (should they occur) are similar.

Of interest are our laboratory investigations that show that a change in the proportion of cells containing a certain marker may be associated with a change in the proportion of cells demonstrating other markers. We have noted that the increase in [^{3}H]TdR-labeled cells is accompanied by a decrease in those demonstrating ER.

Another justification for perioperative therapy is based on the contention of Goldie and Coldman (1979) that as a tumor cell population increases there is an ever-expanding number of drug-resistant phenotypic variants that become more difficult to eradicate. Consequently, combinations of non-cross-resistant drugs should be administered when a tumor population contains as few cells as possible. The Goldie somatic mutation theory seems to provide an alternative and independent explanation to that evoking cell kinetic principles as the basis for drug resistance. The two are not, however, mutually exclusive. With the growth of a tumor, not only are the absolute numbers of resistant cells increased but so is the percentage of resistant cells in the total cell population. The latter is presumed to occur because resistant phenotypes not only multiply as a result of their own intrinsic growth rates but as a consequence of the addition of new mutations from the pool of nonresistant (sensitive) cells (Goldie 1982). As a consequence of the enhanced proliferation of cells following tumor removal, it becomes more likely that the number of resistant phenotypes will increase in the metastatic population. Thus, appropriate perioperative therapy should not only destroy cells made more sensitive by their kinetic alteration but also prevent cell proliferation and so prevent an increase in resistant cells.

A third justification for the use of perioperative therapy relates to repeated observations that surgical manipulations result in "showers" of circulating tumor cells (Fisher and Turnbull 1955; Moore et al. 1957; Roberts et al. 1962). It has been reported that the presence of such cells is *not* related to patient outcome (Engell 1959; Ritchie and Webster 1961; Salsbury 1975). Examination of the studies providing evidence fur such a conclusion, however, reveals that they could not have determined what the consequences of finding circulating cells might be. Insufficient patients with too short a follow-up time were inappropriately analyzed. Most important, outcome was related to the presence or absence of circulating tumor cells without regard for other variables that could have influenced prognosis.

Findings from two clinical trials employing perioperative chemotherapy have provided evidence to indicate that there may be a benefit from such therapy. Our own (Fisher and Fisher 1968) employing thiotepa on the day of surgery and for two successive days thereafter demonstrated an improvement in both disease-free survival and survival in some patients – the first evidence indicating the worth of adjuvant chemotherapy. A Scandinavian trial (Nissen-Meyer et al. 1978) in which cyclophosphamide was administered for six consecutive days starting on the day of operation also indicated an advantage for treated patients.

Since such therapy is apt to neutralize only events that are transient, i. e., cells disseminated and kinetic alterations occurring during the perioperative period, one may conjecture how much more beneficial such treatment will be than conventional treatment given a few weeks to a month following operation. Is that lead time apt to alter significantly an outcome more likely determined by events prior to operation? Despite speculations, a trial of perioperative therapy is likely to provide more definitive biological information relative to human neoplasms than will additional *in vitro* and *in vivo* models. If it is revealed from a study that has truly been a contest (a proper evaluation) that there is no benefit to the use of perioperative therapy, then it may be concluded that the biological consequences of primary tumor removal or of circulating tumor cells released at the time of operation are not likely to be of clinical significance and that further research in that aspect of metastasis should be diminished or redirected. Current biological concepts will then need to be modified or abandoned.

Acknowledgement. Supported by Public Health Serveice Grants from the National Cancer Institute (NCI-U10-CA-12027 and NCI U10-CA 34211) and by a grant from the American Cancer Society (ACS-RC-13).

References

Bonadonna G, Valagussa P (1982) Adjuvant therapy of primary breast cancer. In: Carter SK, Gladstein E, Livingston RB (eds) Principles of cancer treatment. McGraw-Hill, New York, pp 315-326

Cooper RG (1969) Combination chemotherapy in hormone resistant breast cancer. Abstract. Proc Am Assoc Cancer Res 10: 15

Engell HC (1959) Cancer cells in the blood. A five to nine year follow-up study. Ann Surg 149: 457-461

Fisher B, Fisher ER (1968) Role of the lymphatic system in dissemination of tumor. In: Lymph and the lymphatic system. Proceedings of the conference on lymph and the lymphatic system, sponsored by Tulane University School of Medicine, and Committee on Shock, of the National Research Council. Thomas, Springfield, Ill, pp 324-347

Fisher B, Ravdin RG, Ausman RK, et al. (1968) Surgical adjuvant chemotherapy in cancer of the breast: results of a decade of cooperative investigation. Ann Surg 168: 337-357

Fisher B, Carbone P, Economou SG, et al. (1975) L-Phenylalanine mustard (L-PAM) in the management of primary breast cancer: a report of early findings. N Eng J Med 292: 117-122

Fisher B, Glass A, Redmond C, et al. (1977) L-Phenylalanine mustard (L-PAM) in the management of primary breast cancer: an update of earlier findings and a comparison with those utilizing L-PAM plus 5-fluorouracil (5-FU). Cancer 39: 2883-3903

Fisher B, Redmond C, Fisher ER, et al. (1980) The contribution of recent NSABP clinical trials of primary breast cancer therapy to an understanding of tumor biology - an overview of findings. Cancer 46: 1009-1025

Fisher B, Gunduz N, Saffer EA (1983) Influence of the interval between primary tumor removal and chemotherapy on kinetics and growth of metastases. Cancer Res 43: 1488-1492

Fisher ER, Turnbull RB Jr (1955) Cytologic demonstration and significance of tumor cells in the mesenteric venous blood in patients with colorectal carcinoma. Surg Gynecol Obstet 100: 102-108

Goldie JH (1982) Drug resistance and chemotherapeutic strategy. In: Owens AH Jr, Doffey DS, Baylin SB (eds) Tumor cell heterogeneity: origins and implications. Academic, New York, pp 115-125

Goldie JH, Coldman AS (1979) A mathematical model for relating the drug sensitivity of tumors to their spontaneous mutation rate. Cancer Treat Rep 63: 1727-1730

Greenspan EM (1966) Combination cytotoxic chemotherapy in advanced disseminated breast cancer. Mt Sinai J Med (NY) 33: 1-26

Gunduz N, Fisher B, Saffer EA (1979) Effect of surgical removal on the growth and kinetics of residual tumor. Cancer Res 39: 3861-3865

Moore GE, Sanberg AA, Schulbarg JR (1957) Clinical and experimental observations of the occurrence and fat of tumor cells in the bloodstream. Ann Surg 146: 580-587

Nissen-Meyer R et al. (1978) Surgical adjuvant chemotherapy. Results with one short course with cyclophosphamide after mastectomy for breast cancer. Cancer 41: 2088-2098

Ritchie AC, Webster DR (1961) Tumor cells in the blood. In: Begg RW, Ham A, Leblond CP, Noble RL, Rossiter RJ (eds) Proceedings of the fourth Canadian Cancer Conference, 1961. Academic, New York, pp 225-236

Roberts S, Jonasson O, Long L, McGrew EA, McGrath R, Cole WH (1962) Relationship of cancer cells in the circulating blood to operation. Cancer 15: 232-240

Salsbury AJ (1975) The significance of the circulating cancer cell. Cancer Treat Rev 2: 55-72

Schiffer LM, Braunschweiger PG, Stragand JJ (1978) Tumor cell population kinetics following noncurative treatment. Antibiot Chemother 23: 148-156

Simpson-Herren L, Sanford AH, Holmquist JP (1976) Effects of surgery on the cell kinetics of residual tumor. Cancer Treat Rep 60: 1749-1760

Factors Affecting the Development of Permanent Drug Resistance and Its Impact upon Neoadjuvant Chemotherapy

A. J. Coldman and J. H. Goldie

Division of Epidemiology, Biometry and Occupational Oncology, Cancer Control Agency of British Columbia, 600 West 10th Avenue, Vancouver, B.C., V5Z 4E6, Canada

Introduction

Resistance is a general term describing the insensitivity of tumors to treatment. A large amount of research has gone into classifying various biological mechanism which can give rise to resistance to chemotherapy. Various mechanisms have been recognized. Some have been found to operate at the cellular level and some have been found to be due to tumor architecture or location. The importance of each mechanism in explaining the insensitivity of human tumors to chemotherapy is not known, and may vary from site to site. However, the general implications of each mechanism is important and merits detailed investigation.

One mechanism which is important and which can be analyzed mathematically is the spontaneous acquisition of resistance to chemotherapy. This process is believed to arise via specific random alterations in the genetic material which are then preserved at mitosis and which confer either specific or general resistance to chemotherapeutic agents. A significant amount of research with in vitro modeling systems has demonstrated the existence of this mechanism, and genetic changes associated with this form of resistance have been demonstrated (Ling 1982).

The Model

Previously we, and others, have mathematically modeled this process and have made various deductions regarding the consequences of this process on the treatment of human and animal malignancy (Goldie and Coldman 1979; Coldman and Goldie 1983). These models made the following assumptions:

1. Sensitive stem cells spontaneously mutate to a state of permanent drug resistance with a fixed probability α, per division, where α is a function of the drug dose, the drug type, and the malignancy. α is frequently referred to as the mutation rate.
2. Sensitive and resistant stem cells divide and grow at the same rate.
3. Each cell is capable of unlimited proliferation.

Using these assumptions it is possible to calculate the mean number of chemoresistant cells as a function of the mutation rate and the tumor size. Although the mean number of resistant cells is important, the presence of any resistant cells is, according to this model, sufficient to cause therapeutic failure. Therefore, a more interesting quantity is the probability that no resistant cells are present. Assuming that no resistant cells are present initially, this probability starts at unity and decreases monotonically to zero. From this it may

Recent Results in Cancer Research. Vol 103

be seen that smaller tumor burdens are less likely to have resistant cells and thus, other things being equal, are more likely to be cured. This relationship gives support to the concept of neoadjuvant therapy.

However, not every cell is capable of unlimited proliferation and tumors are believed to be stem cell systems similar to several normal tissue systems (Steel 1977). In this system cells are partitioned by their proliferative potential into (1) stem cells, those capable of unlimited proliferation; (2) transitional cells, those capable of limited proliferation; and (3) end cells, which are capable of no proliferation.

The assumption that all cells are stem cells may be relaxed by using birth and death processes, where stem cells may divide to form either two new stem cells (birth) or two transitional cells (death) (Goldie an Coldman 1983; Coldman et al. 1985; Day 1984). This model for tumor growth has been previously discussed elsewhere (MacKillop et al. 1983), as have its implications for the therapy of human malignancy (Goldie and Coldman 1983; Coldman et al. 1985). However, it is not clear that all stem cell systems behave in this way and in some systems it has been postulated (Potten et al. 1978; Vogel et al. 1969) that stem cells divide to form either two new stem cells (birth) or a single transitional cell and a single stem cell (renewal). These two models have widely different implications for the development of metastasis, clonal evolution, and other important clinical variables. However, we will confine ourselves here to the consideration of resistance. This may be modeled

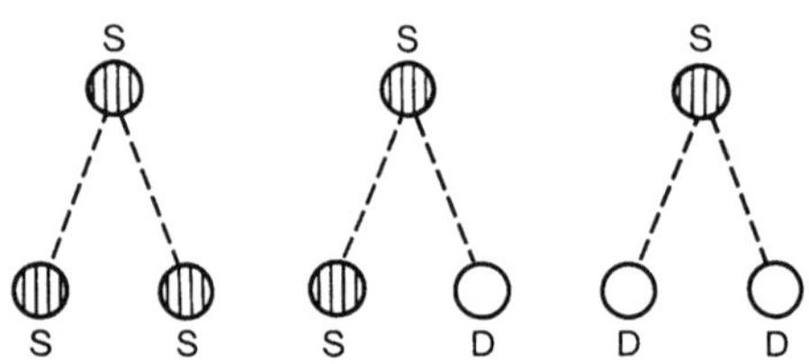

Fig. 1. The possible products of stem cell *(S)* division. They represent, *from left to right,* births, renewals, and deaths

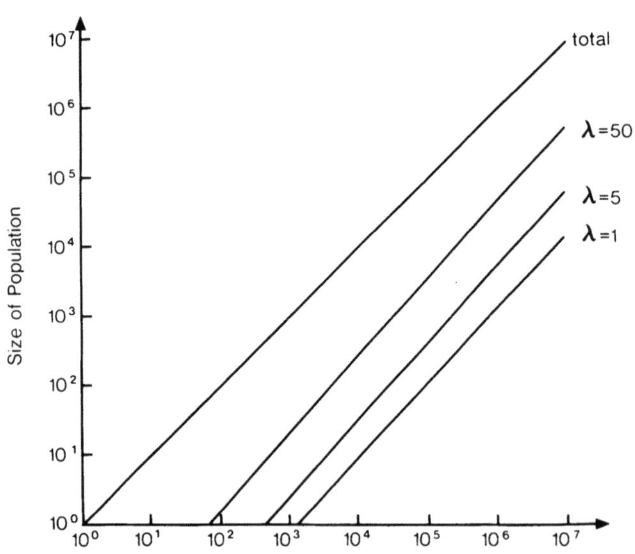

Fig. 2. Plot of the expected number of resistant stem cells as a function of the total number of stem cells for three different rates of growth. It can be seen that as λ increases (rate of growth decreases) the mean number of resistant cells increases

mathematically by considering three rates, *b*, *c*, and *d*, which are the birth rate, the renewal rate, and the death rate respectively. Three types of division are depicted in Fig. 1. Thus a model for $c=0$ would be one where only births and deaths occur, and one for which $d=0$ would be one for which only births and renewals occur. Using a general model we can thus judge the effects of varying of these parameters (*b*, *c*, and *d*) independently. In attempting to use this growth model in real neoplasms, it is necessary to relate *b*, *c*, and *d* to physically measurable quantities. The sum $(b+c+d)$ is the rate at which the stem cells are dividing, so that this quantity is determined from the intermitotic interval. It can be shown that for this model of tumor growth the mean net growth rate is proportional to $b-d$ (MacKillop et al. 1983). For a specific tumor we would equate $b-d$ to the growth rate and examine the effect of varying the parameters *b*, *c*, and *d* on the development of resistance.

The constraints on the values of the parameters, *b*, *c*, and *d* are mostly easily expressed in terms of the quantity λ, where $\lambda = \frac{\text{doubling time of the tumor}}{\text{intermitotic time of the stem cells}}$. Using these constraints there is a relatively narrow range of values of *b*, *c*, and *d* which are permitted. The two extremes of this variation are characterized by the conditions $c=0$ and by $d=0$. The mathematical formula for the mean number of resistant cells using this growth model is given in Appendix A. Figure 2 shows the effect that λ has on the expected number of resistant cells. From this figure it may be seen that as the growth rate slows the expected number of resistant cells increases for a given number of stem cells. After fixing λ and assuming a constant cell division rate the actual values of *b*, *c*, and *d* do not affect the mean number of resistant cells.

Figure 3 shows the effect on the probability of no persistent resistant stem cells, that is the probability that any such cells can grow to cause recurrence. It has been previously shown that for $c=0$ that λ has no effect on this probability. This arises because greater λ implies slower growth rates and thus a greater death rate *d*. There is therefore a greater probability that the cells will spontaneously die out. For the case $d=0$, the probability is strongly dependent on the growth rate, with resistance appearing at smaller sizes in slower

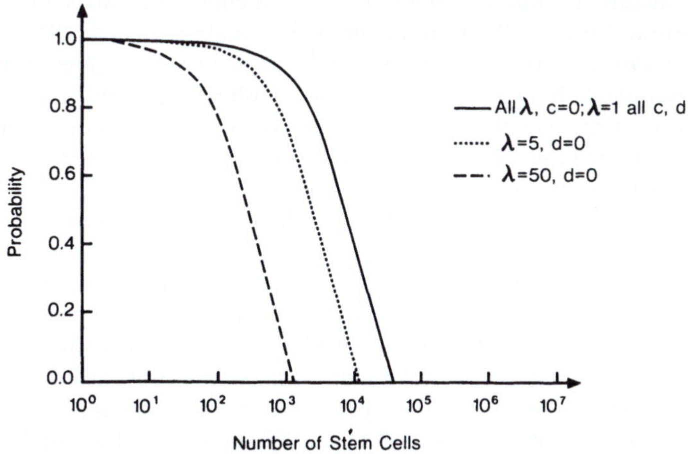

Fig. 3. Probability of no persistent resistent stem cells plotted as a function of stem cell compartment size. The *solid line* indicates the probability curve for all values of λ when $c=0$. The *light dashed* and *heavy dashed lines* plot the probability for $\lambda=5$ and $\lambda=50$ respectively when $d=0$. Thus for $d=0$ decreasing the growth rate (increasing λ) tends to bring about the earlier development of resistant cells which will persist to cause treatment failure

growing tumors. However, the overall shape of these curves is unchanged from the most basic model but it is merely their "location" which is shifted. The formulae for the curves in Fig. 3 are also given in Appendix A.

If we assume that persisting resistant cells imply chemotherapeutic failure and vice versa, then the probability of no resistant cells is equivalent to the probability that the tumor is curable. Thus under this simplifying assumption the long-term cure rate of the tumor fixes the location of the curve (of the probability of no persistent resistant cells) when the pretreatment stem cell burden is known. If the time of commencing treatment is advanced the effect is to move the reference point for the treatment. Since the tumor is smaller et earlier times this implies, because of the shape of the curve, that it will generally be more curable.

Examination of these curves (i.e., Fig. 3) shows that they may be generally partitioned into three regions:

1. A region of high curability where the curve is relatively flat
2. A region of intermediate curability where the curve changes rapidly as a function of tumor size
3. A region of low curability where the curve is flat

An alternate way of partitioning the curve is in terms of its slope at different stem cell compartment sizes. As the curve can only decrease with increasing size of the stem cell compartment, the slope is always negative. Then the three regions may be classified as:

1. A region of high curability with small or little slope
2. A region of intermediate curability with large negative slope
3. A region of low curability with little or no slope

Therefore factors which affect the slope of this curve will directly influence the likely effect of advancing the time of chemotherapy.

Another assumption we have made is that the mutation rate α is fixed for a specific tumor type. This assumption is compatible with much evidence available for passaged animal tumors; however, these represent genetic lines which have undergone considerable amounts of selection on factors such as stability of growth and cloning efficiency. Spontaneous human tumors show much variation in these properties and it does not seem unreasonable to expect that variations in other properties, such as the mutation rates to drug resistance, may also be seen. The effect of differences in mutation rates in relationship to treatment sequencing has been examined elsewhere (Day 1984); we will examine its effect on treatment scheduling.

In order to examine mathematically the effects of variations in α it is first necessary to model this variation. One way in which this may be done is by choosing a set of discrete values for the mutation rate and examining their effect (Day 1984). However, this method is generally not mathematically simple and requires considerable computation. A more comprehensive method is to consider α to have a probability distribution which is equivalent to defining probabilities that α will take on any particular value. If the probability distribution known as the conjugate is chosen, then the mathematical form of the solution is comparatively simple. It is then possible to see how the variability in α influences the clinical effect of advancing the time of chemotherapy. In this case the conjugate is known as the beta distribution (Fig. 4).

In attempting to assess the effect of the distribution of α upon the therapy of clinical disease, it is necessary to vary the parameters in a way such that the overall curability of the tumor is not affected. We do this since the curability is an observed quantity and in

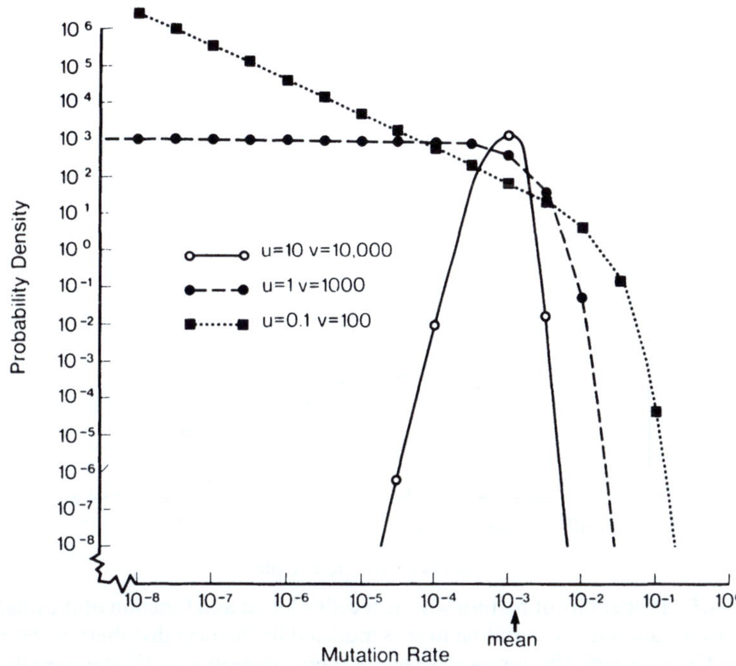

Fig. 4. This plots the beta distribution for three different values of the pair of parameters *u, v.* Each distribution is chosen to have a mean value of approximately 10^{-3}. The *solid* line represents a distribution where the variation in α is small (i.e., standard deviation < mean). The *circled dashed line* represents a case where the variation in α is moderate (standard deviation = mean). The *boxed dashed line* represents a case where the variation is large (standard deviation > mean)

wishing to examine the effect of a theoretical mechanism we cannot change the known characteristics of the system. Figure 5 shows the effect of various choices for the beta distribution, and therefore variations in α, on the probability of no resistant cells in the stem cell compartment. In this example we have required that there be a 25% change of no resistant stem cells for a tumor burden of 10^4 stem cells. It can be seen that the curability at different tumor burdens does not vary greatly as long as the mean mutation rate remains close to that value that it would take if it were not permitted to vary. However, when the mean is far from this value then the probability of no persistent resistance curve can take quite different shapes. Therefore, the slope of the curve, which determines the effect advancing the time of treatment, will vary with the distribution of α. This implies that it is not sufficient just to know the current cure rate to estimate accurately the increase in cures likely to be achieved by earlier chemotherapy because many curves pass through a single point. This contrasts with simpler models where only a single curve passes through each point on the graph of probability versus tumor stem cell compartment size. However, advancing the time of chemotherapy is always advantageous; it is the magnitude of the benefit that will depend on the inherent variation in the mutation rates.

As previously noted, the growth rates of spontaneous tumors is known to vary greatly. Therefore it is possible to analyze the effect of variations in the growth rate in a way analogous to that for examining variations in the mutation rate. However, this analysis is somewhat more complex; since as we have previously shown fixing the growth rate does not uniquely specify the parameters *b, c,* and *d.* Therefore, even for fixed growth rates there is

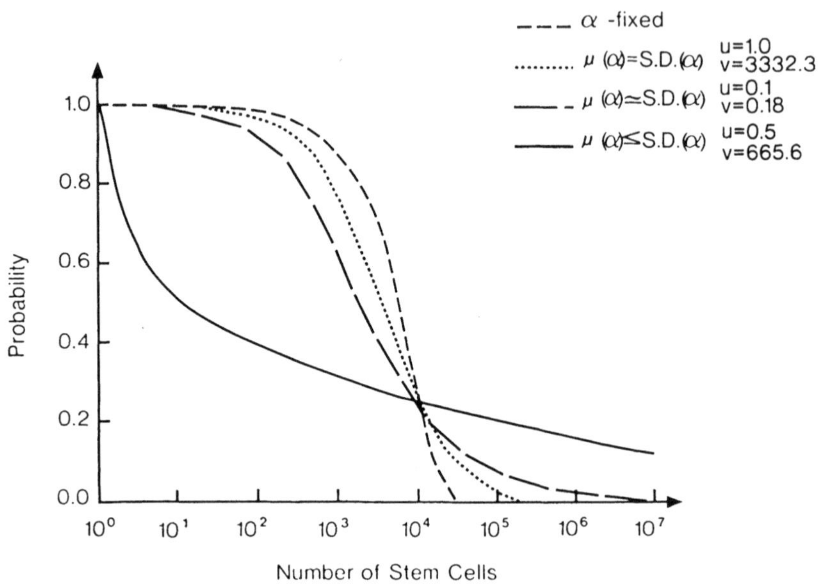

Fig. 5. Probability of no resistant stem cells plotted as a function of the total number of stem cells for various amounts of variation in α as modeled by the beta distribution. *From right to left (in the upper half of the graph)* the curves represent: (1) no variation in α, (2) standard deviation of α = mean of α, (3) standard deviation of $\alpha >$ mean of α, and (4) standard deviation of $\alpha \gg$ mean of α. Each curve is required to yield a 25% probability of no resistant cells for a stem cell burden of 10^4 cells

a substantial latitude for variations in the parameters and when variability in growth rates is considered, this is increased.

An Example

Breast cancer is receiving particular attention as a human malignancy in which the neoadjuvant approach may be tested. This interest, and the relatively extensive data available on the tumor, make it a suitable subject to examine the effect of some of these tumor characteristics on the outcome of therapy. If we assume that all chemotherapeutic failures are a result of mutations to resistance, then it is possible to assess the maximum effect that advancing the time of chemotherapy would have in overcoming this problem. This is, of course, not necessarily the maximum effect which advancing the time of chemotherapy may have, since other factors influencing treatment failure (or possibly potentiating effects) may be more sensitive to this change in timing.

Unfortunately, as in most other mathematical modeling of biological data, it is necessary to make some simplifying assumptions. We will assume that within each tumors' subgroup (defined by nodal and menopausal status) the parameters *b, c,* and *d* are fixed and thus that tumor and cellular doubling times are fixed within these groups. We will assume that within each subgroup every member will have the same preoperative tumor burden. With this assumption it is then possible to calculate the likelihood that a postoperative tumor burden will contain no resistant cells as a function of the mutation rate and the residual burden. It is well accepted that the postoperative tumor burden for breast cancer is highly variable and this will be taken into account using estimates of residual tumor bur-

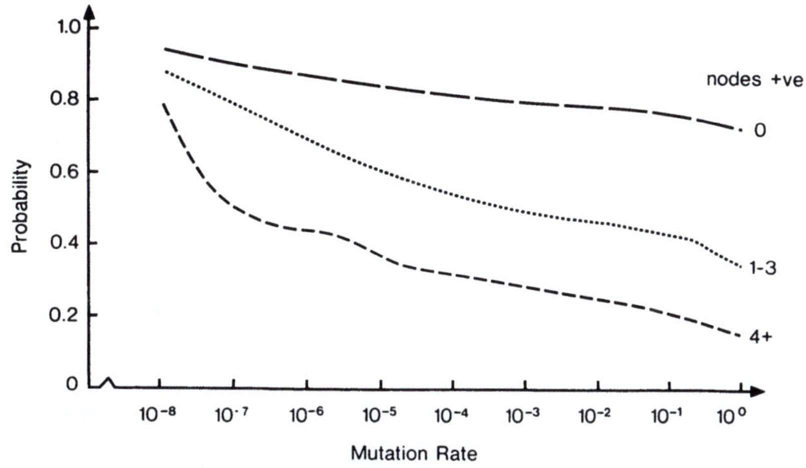

Fig. 6. Probability of no resistant cells plotted as a function of the mutation rate to drug resistance (assumed fixed) for women with premenopausal breast cancer in either of the three nodal groups. The analysis uses the estimates of residual tumor burden derived by Skipper (1979) using the data of Valagussa et al. (1978) The slope of these curves is determined jointly by the proportion of surgical cures and the estimated amount of residual tumor in those not cured surgically. This analysis would imply that although moderately active agents may be expected to have some effect, large increases in the cure rate will require the use of drugs with a low mutation rate

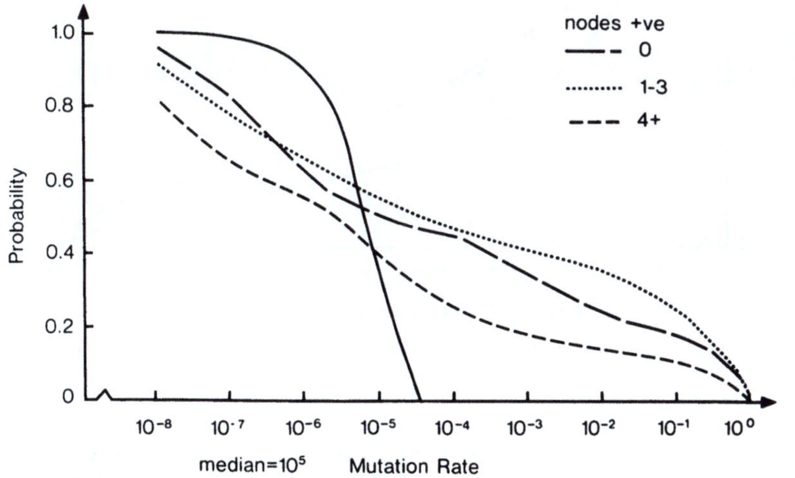

Fig. 7. The same analysis as that in Fig. 6 for the surgical failures alone. The *bold line* indicates the probability of no resistant cells curve appropriate if we were to approximate the frequency distribution of residual tumor by its median

den produced by Skipper (1979), using data collected by Valagussa et al. (1978) on women who received only surgical treatment for their breast cancer.

Figure 6 shows the probability that there will be no resistant cells as a function of the mutation rate for premenopausal disease. Here it has been assumed that 10-year disease-free survival corresponds to cure and that the postoperative tumor burden in this case is zero (Skipper 1979). These figures show the slope of these curves for various nodal in-

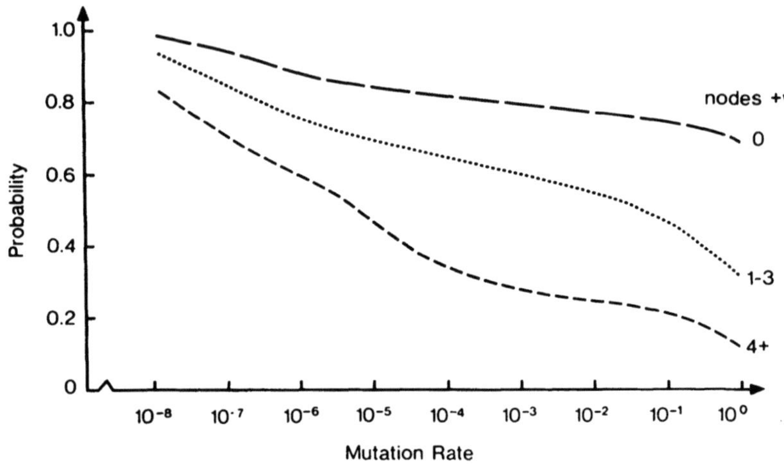

Fig. 8. A similar analysis to that in Fig. 6 for postmenopausal disease

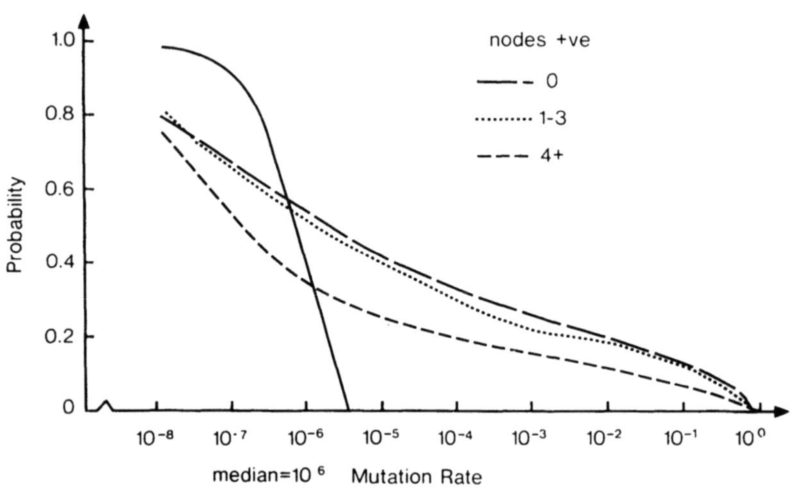

Fig. 9. Again a similar analysis to that in Fig. 7 for postmenopausal disease

volvement groups is quite low. We may use these figures to infer the effect of advancing the time of chemotherapy on the likelihood that resistance will be present. This may be done because the probability of no resistance is a function of the product of the mutation rate and the tumor size (see Appendix A). The effect of reducing N is the same as reducing α by a similar proportion, that is the effect of a single log reduction in the tumor at the time of chemotherapy by advancing the time of chemotherapy is equivalent, in its effect on resistance, to a single log reduction in the mutation rate of the treatment. Figure 7 gives the results of the same analysis applied to the surgical failures alone. This analysis suggests that any advancing of the time of therapy will have similar effects on the treatment failures in each of the three nodal groups if the mutation rates do not vary systematically between these groups. For comparison a curve is also included which would be appropriate if, rather than the observed distribution of postoperative tumor burdens, each surgical failure had a burden which was equal to median burden. From this it is clear that it is necessary to consider the full distribution of residual tumor burden; otherwise, the use of the median burden gives an erroneous picture. Figures 8 and 9 present the results of a similar analysis for postmenopausal disease. Comparison of the results for pre- and postmenopausal disease shows that for each nodal group the slope is similar for both pre- and postmenopausal disease. However, the estimated growth rate of premenopausal breast cancer is greater than that of postmenopausal breast cancer and thus earlier chemotherapy will have a lesser effect in decreasing the likelihood of resistance for post- as compared with premenopausal disease. This emphasizes the most obvious conclusion which may be made, that other things being equal more rapidly growing tumors are more likely to benefit from the prompt application of chemotherapy.

Using this theory and data it is possible to estimate the likely effects of advancing the timing of chemotherapy on long-term curability. These calculations suggest that long-term cures will be increased by approximately 3% for premenopausal disease and 2% for postmenopausal cancer, when comparing 28-day postsurgical therapy with therapy 7 days preoperative. This calculation assumes that the total effect of neoadjuvant therapy is in its effect in preventing drug resistance and that the date of surgery has not been altered. Its possible effect on other factors such as presurgical tumor consolidation has not been considered and these may either increase of decrease the magnitude of the likely gains. Intervals between neoadjuvant and adjuvant therapy of less than 35 days will have correspondingly lesser effects. The preceding calculations of the likely effect of advancing the time of first treatment probably underestimate the true effect as they are based upon an analysis (MacKillop et al. 1983) which assumes fixed doubling times of all premenopausal and all postmenopausal tumors. Ignoring the likely variation in postsurgical regrowth rates will tend to exaggerate the variation in postsurgical tumor burden, which will cause the effect of advancing the time of treatment to be underestimated.

Interestingly, the effect of variations in the mutation rate on this analysis is not pronounced and will not be presented here. We noted before that its effect was to diminish likely improvements due to earlier scheduling when considering tumors of a fixed size. However, in the case of postsurgical breast cancer, the size distribution is of sufficient variability to dilute any effects attributable to variations in the mutation rate.

Conclusion

Factors affecting tumor growth have been shown to influence the development of drug resistance. Any factor which increases the rate at which stem cells divide per unit of net tumor growth is shown to increase the rate at which drug-resistant cells accumulate. The process of stem cell division, involving births, renewals, and deaths, cannot be discerned directly by observing the intermitotic interval and the growth rate of the tumor. This uncertainty coupled with variations in growth rates and mutation rates between tumors make it difficult to predict the likely variation in resistance between tumors and thus the influence which these variations will have on the effect of the neoadjuvant approach. Nevertheless, despite this uncertainty it is clear that earlier treatment reduces the likelihood for resistance to emerge and the clinical usefulness of this approach will await the outcome of clinical trials.

Acknowledgement. This research was supported, in part, by the British Columbia Health Care Research Foundation.

Appendix A

It is straightforward to show that the expected number of resistant stem cells, $m(t)$, is approximately given by $m(t)=(\alpha_1 b+\alpha_2 c)(b-d)^{-1} N(t) \ln N(t)$, where $N(t)(N(0)=1)$ is the total number of stem cells, α_1 is the mutation rate to resistant for stem cell births, and α_2 is the mutation rate to resistant for stem cell renewals.

In the absence of information to the contrary, it seems reasonable to assume $\alpha_2=\frac{1}{2}\alpha_1$. From this we can easily show $m(t)=\frac{\alpha_1}{2}(1+\lambda) N(t) \ln N(t)$, which is the same for all parameter choices b, c, and d which result in equal growth rates (i.e., the same λ).

The probability of no mutations to resistance, $P(t)$, may easily be shown to be $P(t)=\exp\left\{-\frac{\alpha_1}{2}(1+\lambda)(N(t)-1)\right\}$, which is again identical for all b, c, d which result in the same growth rate.

The probability that any resistant cells will persist to cause failure $P_F(t)$ has previously been shown (Coldman et al. 1985) to be given by $P_F(t)=\exp\{-\alpha_1(N(t)-1)\}$, when $c=0$. However, when $d=0$, $P_F(t)=P(t)$ and thus this quantity will vary with the growth rate.

We may write $P_F(t)$ generally as $P_F(t)=\{-\alpha'(N(t)-1)\}$, where α' is a function of α_1, α_2, b, c, and d. For $\alpha' \ll 1$, $P_F(t) \simeq (1-\alpha')^{N(t)-1}$

If we assume that for any tumor α' does not vary in time and model the variation (between tumors) in α' using a beta distribution $\beta(u, v)$ then it may be shown that

$$E[P_F(t)]=\prod_{i=1}^{N(t)-1}\left(\frac{v+i-1}{u+v+i-1}\right).$$

References

Coldman AJ, Goldie JH (1983) A model for the resistance of tumor cells to cancer chemotherapeutic agents. Math Biosci 65: 291-307

Coldman AJ, Goldie JH, Ng V (1985) The effect of cellular differentiation of the development of permanent drug resistance. Math Biosci (in press)

Day R (1984) A tumor growth model with applications to treatment policy and protocol choice. PhD Thesis in Biostatistics, Harvard School of Public Health

Goldie JB, Coldman AJ (1979) A mathematic model for relating the drug sensitivity of tumors to their spontaneous mutation rate. Cancer Treat Rep 63: 1727-1733

Goldie JH, Coldman AJ (1983) A quantitative model for multiple levels of drug resistance in clinical tumours. Cancer Treat Rep 67: 923-931

Ling V (1982) Genetic basis of drug resistance in mammalian cells. In: Bruchovsky N, Goldie J (eds) Drug and hormone resistance in neoplasia, vol 1. CRC Press, Boca Raton, pp 1-19

MacKillop WJ, Ciampi A, Till JE, Buick RN (1983) A stem cell model of human tumor growth: implication for tumor cell clonogenic assays. JNCI 70: 9-16

Potten CS, Hume WJ, Reid P, Cairns J (1978) The segregation of DNA in epithelial stem cells. Cell 15: 899-906

Skipper H (1979) Repopulation rates of breast cancer cells after mastectomy (judged from breakpoints in remission - duration curves). Booklet 12, Southern Research Institute, Birmingham

Steel GG (1977) Growth kinetics of tumours. Clarendon, Oxford, p 218

Valagussa P, Bonnadonna G, Veronesi U (1978) Patterns of relapse and survival in operable breast carcinoma with positive and negative axillary nodes. Tumori 64: 241-258

Vogel H, Niewisch H, Matioli E (1969) Stochastic development of stem cells. J Theor Biol 22: 249-270

Impact of Preoperative Chemotherapy for the Surgeon

R. M. Baird and P. A. Rebbeck

Department of Surgery, University of British Columbia, Vancouver, B.C., Canada

The utilization of chemotherapeutic drugs during the pre- or perioperative period has very significant theoretical and practical implications for the surgeon. Many of the drugs which are used have marked systemic effects and may influence operative morbidity and mortality. In particular, specific alterations in wound healing must be considered. The organization and administration of multimodality therapy must also be taken into account. Chemotherapeutic agents may be administered by the surgeon if he or she is experienced in the use of these drugs, but most frequently patients will be handled by the team approach which will include the surgeon, medical oncologist, and radiation oncologist.

Cancer diagnosis may be confirmed by open biopsy or fine-needle aspiration cytology. Cytological techniques have only recently gained wide acceptance and one must remain cautious in relying entirely on this diagnostic method. As cytopathologists gain more experience, the accuracy of this technique is becoming increasingly reliable, but the surgeon must also be cautious about the possibility of a false-positive report in a patient who is to be administered a potentially toxic drug. In breast cancer, the false-positive rate in most reported series is now well under 1% (Pontifex and Suen 1981; Frable 1983), and in our opinion it is valid to administer chemotherapeutic drugs to patients in whom the diagnosis has been obtained by this technique alone. In a personal series of 84 breast cancer cases no false-positive cytology was observed. However, it is the responsibility of the surgeon to ensure that the cytological reports they obtain have a high degree of accuracy.

A continuing internal review within ones own institution to monitor the accuracy of cytological reports is important. There must be good communication between the surgeon and cytopathologist in order to correlate the clinical, mammographic, and cytological findings. In many instances it is desirable that the slides by reviewed by more than one cytopathologist.

Frequently the surgeon will be the patient's first oncological consultant. The surgeon must therefore be knowledgeable with the types of drugs used and their mode of administration, complications, and possible side effects. It will frequently by the surgeon's responsibility to obtain informed consent for neoadjuvant chemotherapy. The surgeon must be prepared to organize the administration of preoperative chemotherapy prior to the patient's admission to hospital and to time the surgery accordingly. At present, however, pharmacokinetic data are insufficient and the timing of preoperative drug administration remains empirical. Hopefully, drug administration related to surgery will become less empirical in the future.

Chemotherapy agents have specific systemic effects which must be considered when major surgery is to be undertaken (Shamberger et al. 1981; Ferguson 1982). Thrombocytopenia is a frequent complication, but providing that platelet counts are carefully monitored, difficulty with hemostasis should not be a perioperative problem. There may also

Recent Results in Cancer Research. Vol 103

be impairment of liver function, either from the drugs or from the malignancy. Providing that liver function tests are within reasonable levels, the surgery should not be adversely affected.

Many malnourished patients may have this condition aggravated by the preoperative chemotherapy. Although protein depletion and other specific nutritional deficiencies such as ascorbic acid deficiency do alter wound healing, there is seldom significant impairment unless severe malnutrition is present. If the nutritional state is poor it can be improved by a preoperative course of parenteral or enteral nutrition.

Leukopenia associated with chemotherapy increases the susceptibility to infection (Simpson and Ross 1972; Kraft et al. 1979). If the surgical wound is sterile, it will heal in a normal manner. However, if the operative field is contaminated, such as in head and neck or bowel surgery, extra caution must be exercised to prevent wound infection and appropriate prophylactic antibiotics must be used.

Anemia may be associated with volume deficits or malnutrition (Heughan et al. 1974) or may be due to chemotherapy. Patients with significant chronic obstructive lung disease or coronary artery disease must have their anemia corrected prior to elective surgery. Providing that the tissues remain adequately oxygenated, anemia does not adversely affect wound healing.

Although neoadjuvant chemotherapy trials are relatively recent and the appropriate safety studies preliminary, many patients undergoing surgery have received chemotherapeutic agents prior to surgery. Ferrara et al. (1982) reviewed the results of patients receiving chemotherapy who required emergency surgery, and observed that surgery was generally well tolerated.

Finn et al. (1980) have analyzed 175 patients with disseminated or locally advanced cancer who were receiving chemotherapy and required surgery. Complications such as pneumonia, wound infections, and wound dehiscence were seen in 5.9% of the cases, but the overall mortality was only 2.2%. The complications and mortality were not unusually high when the advanced state of malignancy and the magnitude of surgery are considered. With current sophisticated operative care, morbidity and mortality rates can be kept at an acceptable level, not only in patients with advanced malignant disease but also in those receiving aggressive chemotherapy prior to surgery.

Anesthetics and chemotherapeutic agents may interact with potentially toxic effects. The Ludwig Breast Cancer Study Group (1983) noted, in patients receiving cyclophosphamide, methotrexate, and 5-fluorouracil within 36 of mastectomy, that complications were significantly increased in the treated group. In this study, four deaths occurred among 327 patients. The causes of death included pneumonia, renal failure, myelosuppression, wound infection, septic shock, and pulmonary embolus. Toxicity was more frequent in patients over 50 years of age. The authors were of the opinion that the combination of nitrous oxide and methotrexate was hazardous and suggested the use of leucovorin with methotrexate in patients anesthetized with nitrous oxide. Although the report of the Ludwig Group is of concern, similar complications have not been the experience of other groups. Pharmacological information is inadequate at this time specifically to implicate this association and further work is required before the combination of methotrexate and nitrous oxide is abandoned.

The information available from clinical studies is sparse, but extensive data are available from animal experiments on the effect of chemotherapeutic agents on wound healing.

The healing of a closed wound is a complex phenomenon which involves three distinct phases. The initial phase of inflammation is characterized by an increase in vascular permeability with an influx of erythrocytes, polymorpholeukocytes, monocytes, and platelets, and deposition of fibrin. Proteolytic enzymes and vasoactive substances are released into the wound and an activated complement system attracts macrophages which clear the inflammatory debris. Chemotherapeutic drugs appear to have very little effect on this phase, although bone marrow depression can affect the influx of leukocytes.

The proliferative phase begins within 4 days and is characterized by neovascularization with fibroblast proliferation and the production of mucopolysaccharides and collagen. This phase lasts up to 4 weeks and may be affected much more drastically by systemic factors than the inflammatory phase may be. The effect of chemotherapeutic agents on RNA and DNA may affect fibroblast proliferation as well as collagen and mucopolysaccharide production. The myofibroblast is of great importance in wound contraction and inhibition of its production or function will significantly affect the healing process.

The last phase, that of maturation, goes on for some months with cross-linkage and alignment of collagen fibers. Any agent affecting collagen metabolism will be harmful at this phase.

In consideration of the effects of any chemotherapeutic agent, several factors need to be considered. Particularly in the neoadjuvant setting the timing of the drug administration is of great importance and in many studies it has not been adequately considered. A drug administered 1 week prior to wounding may have no effect on the wound but when given 4 days postwounding it may produce deleterious effects. The organ undergoing surgery is also important, for delayed or impaired healing of intestinal anastomosis may cause leakage, while delay in the healing of an abdominal incision or a mastectomy wound will be of less significance. Surgery in potentially contaminated areas such as the head and neck, gastrointestinal tract, or the lung will be more adversely affected by drugs reducing the granulocyte counts, with subsequent decreased resistance to infection.

Experimental studies have shown that nitrogen mustard and cyclophosphamide reduce wound breaking strength. The precise mechanism has not been determined but it has been postulated that an inhibition of fibroplasia, or possibly of vasodilatation and subsequent neovascularization, occurs (Ferguson 1982; Fahrat et al. 1958; Cohen et al. 1975). Thiotepa does not appear to inhibit wound healing in experimental animals unless given in massive doses (Fahrat et al. 1958).

Methotrexate inhibits wound healing in the rat when given from day 1 to day 5 but it seems to have little effect when given after day 5. The effect can be reversed with leucovorin rescue (Calnan and Davies 1965).

5-Fluorouracil inhibits abdominal wall healing, but perhaps of more significance is its adverse effects on the healing of colonic anastomosis (Goldman et al. 1965; Staley et al. 1961). Studies on 6-mercaptopurine are controversial and definite conclusions cannot be made at present.

Actinomycin D and bleomycin (Cohen et al. 1975) impair the healing of wounds tested at 3 and 7 days but not at 21 days postinjury. Adriamycin has also been studied extensively (Shamberger et al. 1981), impairing wound healing at doses in the order of the LD_{10}, but at therapeutic doses the impairment is less marked. The effects are most marked when given on day 7 preinjury. When given later at day 7 postinjury, there appear to be no deleterious effects on wound healing. The drug may impair collagen synthesis, for it has been shown that these wounds have decreased collagen content. Concomitant radiotherapy will enhance the adverse effects of Adriamycin. In another study on Adriamycin by Bland et al. (1984), in which the drug was given preoperatively to cachectic animals with tumors, it was noted that the wound tensile strength was decreased in the cachectic but not in the normal animals.

In the mouse, vincristine given on the day of injury does impair wound healing when the wound is tested on the 3rd day following injury. However, on the 7th or 21st day post-injury, wound healing appears to be proceeding normally (Cohen et al. 1975). The transitory nature of the drugs effect may explain why more adverse effects are not evident clinically.

Corticosteroids reduce the normal inflammatory response to wounding with decreased production of granulation tissue and delayed epithelialization. For the patient on long-term high-dose corticosteroids this may be of significance, but if steroids are started postoperatively healing of the wound does not appear to be retarded.

Estrogens and progestatives decrease granuloma formation but the effects appear to be negligible (Peacock and Van Winkle 1976). Anabolic steroids increase tensile strength and accelerate wound contraction (Peacock and Van Winkle 1976). There are no data available as yet on the effect of antiestrogens on wound healing.

A brief review of the animal studies available does emphasize that most of the chemotherapeutic drugs available have deleterious effects on wound healing. The effect varies with the drug dosage and time of administration. When these drugs are utilized in the neoadjuvant setting, the timing of administration is of prime importance. Many experimental studies have not emphasized this aspect adequately.

Fortunately, in the clinical setting, minor inhibition of would healing does not appear to result in significant morbidity. The significance of any impairment in wound healing will vary with the site of the surgery. The most hazardous areas would include the gastrointestinal tract, where impaired healing of a colonic anastomosis could result in a fistula and serious sepsis. But in other areas such as the breast, some delay in healing of the wound will not be of major significance. It has been known for a number of years that clinical complications may occur with neoadjuvant chemotherapy. In an early publication of the NSABP on adjuvant chemotherapy in breast cancer (Cohn et al. 1968) it was noted that local complications occurred more frequently with the 5-fluorouracil group than with the thio-TEPA or untreated control groups. However, the control group had a 40% local complication rate, which is much higher than occurs presently. Breast surgery at that time was more radical than at present; in particular, skin margins were much wider, which probably counts for the high incidence of local recurrence. Another clinical study indicating the potential hazards of neoadjuvant chemotherapy has been reported by Bland et al. (1984). In seven patients with advanced breast cancer receiving three preoperative cycles of Adriamycin at a mean dose of 96.5 mg/cycle, significant complications occurred, with ischemic flap necrosis in five patients. The control group of 20 patients had only two similar complications. The numbers are small but do indicate that Adriamycin may cause significant impairment of wound healing. This report is of particular interest as wound tensile strength was measured. In five melanoma patients receiving 20 mg Adriamycin intravenously with the tourniquet occlusion technique, the primary tumor was excised 6–8 weeks later and at that time the wound tensile strength and wound breaking strength was measured and found to be significantly reduced over the normal.

Postoperative adjuvant therapy has been used with no significant impairment of wound healing (Hubbard et al. 1978; Kardinal and Luce 1977; Shields et al. 1977; Higgins et al. 1971; Ansfield et al. 1969; Hattori et al. 1966). These studies have included breast, ovary, lung, colon, testicular, gastric, and head and neck tumors.

In a series carried out by the authors (Ragaz et al. 1985), 43 patients were treated with cyclophosphamide, methotrexate, and 5-fluorouracil (CMF) prior to definitive breast surgery. No significant impairment of wound healing occurred, infection rates were not altered, and there was no significant alteration in operative morbidity. Similarly, no significant postoperative complications were reported in a group of patients with locally advanced breast cancer receiving preoperative chemotherapy (Morris et al. 1978). Although chemotherapeutic agents clearly affect wound healing in experimental animals, in most clinical studies postoperative mortality due to this condition is infrequent. If used with caution, chemotherapeutic agents in the pre- or perioperative setting is safe. However, clinical studies need close monitoring to avoid the potential hazardous effects of these drugs on the surgical patient.

One concludes from a review of the material available in this field that chemotherapeutic agents do adversely affect wound healing in the experimental animal. Most clinical studies have not shown that chemotherapeutic drugs adversely effect postoperative morbidity. If used with caution, utilization of these drugs in the neoadjuvant setting is safe. It must be stressed that as new agents become available and new combinations are utilized, that further animal studies be done to assess these agents and combinations, and that clinical studies be closely monitored to review the potentially hazardous effects of these drugs on the surgical patient.

References

Ansfield FL, Korbitz BC, Davis HL, Raminez G (1969) Triple drug therapy in testicular tumours. Cancer 24: 442-446

Bland KI, Palin WE et al (1984) Experimental and clinical observations of the effects of cytotoxic chemotherapeutic drugs on wound healing. Ann Surg 199 (6): 782-790

Calnan J, Davies A (1965) The effect of methotrexate (Amethopterin) on wound healing: an experimental study. Br J Cancer 19: 505-212

Cohen SC, Gabelnick HI, Johnson RK et al (1975) Effects of antineoplastic agents on wound healing in mice. Surgery 78: 238-244

Cohn I Jr, Slack NH, Fisher B (1968) Complications and toxic manifestations of surgical adjuvant chemotherapy for breast cancer. Surg Gynecol Obstet 127 (6): 1201-1209

Fahrat SM, Amer NS, Weeks DS et al (1958) Effect of mechlorethamine hydrochloride (nitrogen mustard) on healing of abdominal wounds. Arch Surg 76: 749-753

Falcone RE, Nappi JF (1984) Chemotherapy and wound healing. Surg Clin North Am 64 (4): 779-794

Ferguson MK (1982) The effect of antineoplastic agents on wound healing. Surg Gynecol Obstet 154 (3): 421-429

Ferrara JJ, Martin EW Jr, Carey LC (1982) Morbidity of emergency operations in patients with metastatic cancer receiving chemotherapy. Surgery 92 (4): 605-609

Finn D, Steele G Jr, Osteen RT, Wilson RE (1980) Morbidity and mortality after surgery in patients with disseminated or locally advanced cancer receiving systemic chemotherapy. J Surg Oncol 13: 237-244

Frable WJ (1983) Fine-needle aspiration biopsy: a review. Human Pathol 14: 9-28

Goldman LI, Lowe S, Al-Saleem T (1965) Effect of fluorouracil on intestinal anastomoses in the rat. Arch Surg 98: 303-304

Hattori T, Ito I, Hirata K, Iizuka T, Abe K (1966) Combined treatment in patients with cancer of the stomach: palliative gastrectomy, large does mitomycin-C and bone marrow transplantation. Gann 57: 441-451

Heughan C, Grislis G, Hunt TK (1974) Effect of anemia on wound healing. Ann Surg 179: 163-167

Higgins GA, Dwight RW, Smith JV, Keehn RJ (1971) Fluorouracil as an adjuvant to surgery in carcinoma of the colon. Arch Surg 102: 339-343

Hubbard SM, Barkes P, Young RC (1978) Adriamycin therapy for advanced ovarian carcinoma recurrent after chemotherapy. Cancer Treat Rep 62: 1375-1377

Kardinal CG, Luce JK (1977) Evaluation of hexamethylemelamine and 5-fluorouracil combination in the treatment of advanced ovarian carcinoma. Cancer Treat Rep 61: 1691-1693

Kraft RL, Goldberg NH, Ariyan S (1979) Effect of preoperative high-dose methotrexate and leucovorin rescue on incidence of wound infection in rats. Surg Forum 30: 537-539

Ludwig Breast Cancer Study Group (1983) Toxic effects of early adjuvant chemotherapy for breast cancer. Lancet II: 542-544

Morris DN, Aisner J, Elias EG (1978) Mastectomy as an adjunct to chemoprevention. Arch Sci 113: 282-284

Peacock E, Van Winkle W (1976) Wound repair, 2nd edn. Saunders, Philadelphia

Pontifex AH, Suen KC (1981) Fine needle aspiration diagnosis of breast masses. British Columbia Medical Journal 23: 542-543

Ragaz J, Baird RM, Rebbeck PA, Goldie JH, Coldman AJ, Spinelli JJ (1985) Neo-adjuvant (pre-operative) chemotherapy for breast cancer. Cancer 56: 3-8

Shamberger RC, Devereux DF, Brennan MF (1981) The effect of chemotherapeutic agents on wound healing. Int Adv Surg Oncol 4: 15-58

Shields TW, Humphrey EW, Eastridge CE, Keehn RJ (1977) Adjuvant cancer chemotherapy after resection of carcinoma of the lung. Cancer 40: 2057-2062

Simpson DM, Ross R (1972) The neutrophilic leukocyte in wound repair. A study with anti-neutrophil serum. J Clin Invest 51: 2009-2023

Staley CJ, Trippel OH, Preston FW (1961) Influence of 5-fluorouracil on wound healing. Surgery 49: 450-453

Preoperative (Neoadjuvant) Chemotherapy for Breast Cancer: Outline of the British Columbia Trial

J. Ragaz

Cancer Control Agency of British Columbia, 600 West 10th Avenue,
Vancouver, B.C., V5Z 4E6, Canada

Introduction

The results of the major adjuvant chemotherapy trials show a positive impact of this treatment on the natural history of breast cancer (Jones and Salmon 1984) and, therefore, despite some contrary opinions, adjuvant therapy will likely remain the main form of systemic therapy for newly diagnosed high-risk patients. The number of failure cases after the therapy with conventional adjuvant therapy is, however, still high. In the absence of new curative agents for breast cancer, improvement of scheduling and manipulation of old drugs is the only option left for clinicians to improve survival. Neoadjuvant (preoperative) chemotherapy is an example of such manipulation and its application in the management of breast cancer will be a part of this discussion.

Neoadjuvant therapy can be defined as a systemic treatment given at the earlier possible time after tissue diagnosis of cancer is obtained and before the definitive locoregional therapy is started. According to our definition, the preoperative timing of adjuvant chemotherapy is not the only aspect of this novel treatment. It includes other new trends in adjuvant therapy such as treatment with more intensive systemic combinations consisting of the most effective chemotherapy agents. Neoadjuvant therapy also includes other features, such as a more uniform adoption of conservative surgery, wider use of fine-needle aspiration for obtaining primary diagnosis of cancer and utilization of information from the prechemotherapy assessment of the risk factors in the neoadjuvant staging.

Three aspects of the neoadjuvant treatment will be discussed:

1. Its basic rationale
2. Outline of the British Columbia preoperative adjuvant chemotherapy trial in premenopausal patients with breast cancer
3. Future prospects of neoadjuvant chemotherapy

Rationale

There are several observations from animal experiments (Corbett et al. 1978; Fisher et al. 1983) and from theoretical models (Goldie and Coldman 1979) which point toward benefits of early, as compared with a delayed, timing of chemotherapy used for therapy of most of the tumors. This observation has now been confirmed in human breast cancer. Chemotherapy regimens which fail to alter the natural history of established metastatic disease (delayed treatment) have been shown to cure subsets of patients treated in adjuvant settings (early treatment). It is presently not known whether further reduction of the

Recent Results in Cancer Research. Vol 103

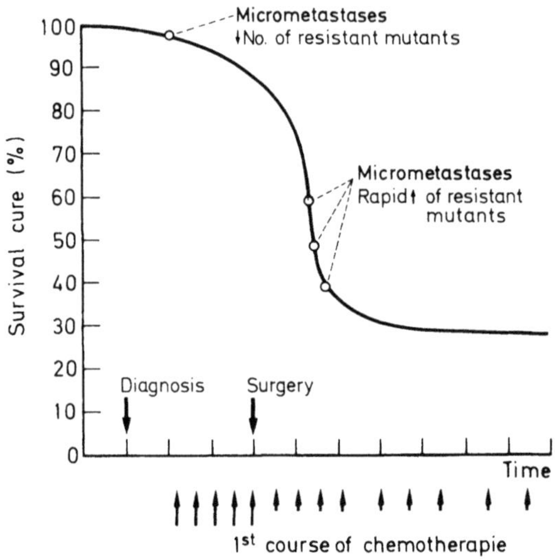

Fig. 1. Correlation of the timing of the first course of adjuvant chemotherapy with the probability survival (see text)

delay time between the diagnosis and the start of adjuvant chemotherapy to the range of days and weeks will result in further improvement but some data (Nissen-Meyer et al. 1978; Jones et al. 1984) indicate that this may be the case. Of importance are several interrelating biological phenomena accompanying development of early subclinical micrometastatic disease. These include, in particular, the resistance and kinetic changes accompanying the surgery. In other parts of this volume, Goldie and Coldman discuss in more detail the significance of resistance and other implications of the somatic mutation theory. We will, therefore, limit our discussion on resistance by pointing only to some of its relevant aspects in connection with the timing of the adjuvant chemotherapy treatment of breast cancer.

Figure 1 outlines the estimated probability percentage for long-term survival of the patients treated with adjuvant chemotherapy. It shows that up to 30% of all patients with breast cancer - those without the micrometastases - can be cured by surgical resection alone. The remaining 65% of cases will have a recurrence and in order to be cured will have to receive some form of systemic treatment, presently represented by adjuvant chemotherapy. The graph shows that as a direct result of accumulation of resistant cells during the delays of starting adjuvant treatment, the probability percentage for cure will rapidly decrease with time. After a certain point the system is incurable with the presently available chemotherapy agents, a situation represented by a plateau of the probability curve. The graph emphasizes that there may be a certain time when the timing of the administration of the first cycle of chemotherapy will be of crucial importance. The delays of the treatment, after this time, as represented by the small arrows, may be of no further importance. The timing of the chemotherapy, therefore, may be of significance only in the pre- or early perioperative period, and delays of more than several weeks or months may not have any further impact.

A review of the literature shows no uniform consensus on the importance of the more minor delays with starting adjuvant chemotherapy. Nissen-Meyer et al. (1978) and Jones et al. (1984) have shown that long as opposed to short delays adversely affect the outcome ($P=0.01$ and 0.02 respectively). On the other hand, the data from the South West Oncology Group (SWOG) (Glucksberg et al. 1982) and from the M.D. Anderson Hospital (Buz-

Table 1. Correlation between the relapse and the mean delay between the diagnosis and the first cycle of LMF chemotherapy (DG-CT-INT). (H.J. Senn, 1985, personal communication)

	Relapse	No Relapse	*P* (one tail)
DG-CT-INT (days)	32	23	0.05
SD	39.14	12	

dar et al. 1982) show that the duration of interval between the diagnosis and start of chemotherapy are of no significance. We have recently analyzed the data from the Ostschweizerische Arbeitsgruppe für klinische Onkologie (OSAKO) study, which were forwarded to us by Senn et al. In the OSAKO trial (Senn et al. 1981), patients with newly diagnosed cancer of the breast were treated with the LMFP (leukeran, methotrexate, fluorouracil, prednisone) chemotherapy regimen (Senn et al. 1981) with or without BCG. The review of the first 117 patients has shown that the mean delay between the diagnosis and the first day of chemotherapy (DT-DT-INT) was 32 days in the relapsing and 23 days in nonrelapsing patients ($P = 0.05$) (see Table 1).

In summary, the question of the significance of delays with instituting postoperative adjuvant chemotherapy is not presently resolved and the outcome of ongoing randomized studies will be of interest (Goldhirsch 1983).

Kinetic Aspects of Preoperative Chemotherapy

Although unpredictable phases of altered spurts of growth of early primary tumor and its micrometastases are suspected, the overall growth pattern of the malignant tumor, according to many investigators, can be best characterized by Gompertzian function. Accordingly, it is expected that along with the expansion of overall tumor cell burden, the growth fraction of the individual cells with exponentially decrease. It is, therefore, expected that noncurative cytoreduction, by means of surgery, chemotherapy, or radiotherapy, may shift the proliferation rate from a flat on to the steep slope of the Gompertzian curve (Ragaz et al. 1985). Noncurative reduction of the tumor cell burden may thus increase the proliferation rate of the surviving malignant cells. Multiple animal experiments have indeed confirmed this observation (Gorelik et al. 1978; Simpson-Herren et al. 1976; DeWyss 1972). Pertinent to the association of the effect of the kinetic changes and the timing of preoperative chemotherapy, several comments can be made. First, on theoretical grounds, the increased cell division in the early postoperative period, in addition to a rapid quantitative expansion of the tumor cell burden, may lead to several phenotypic changes. It is expected that with each cell division involving the genetic mechanisms, the chance for the transition toward pleiotropic resistance to chemotherapy may increase (Coldman personal communication). This suggests that in the early postoperative period the increased growth fraction of the remaining tumor cells, although in theory desirable for an effective cell kill after therapy with certain chemotherapy agents, may, nevertheless, result in a more rapid systemic dissemination very early in the peri- or postoperative period. Of particular concern is the infrequently discussed issue of repopulation and invasion of tumor sanctuaries, which may likely be enhanced after the outburst of the proliferative activity. Thus, a different mechanism of resistance to chemotherapy, further decreasing the chance of cure, will need to be considered.

In summary, the main theoretical benefit of the preoperative chemotherapy is expected to stem from the maximum and fastest reduction of tumor cell burden at the earliest time in the tumor's history. Such an approach may reduce all adverse effects associated with both the delay of starting the chemotherapy treatment as well as with the suspected phenomena following the noncurative surgery.

There is increasing evidence from several biological systems indicating that preoperative chemotherapy is more effective than postoperative treatment. Of interest are observations of Corbett et al. on increase of survival as well as decrease of locoregional recurrence rate after preoperative, as opposed to postoperative, chemotherapy in mice mammary carcinoma (Corbett et al. 1978). Interesting data regarding the dose intensity of preoperative chemotherapy in animal systems come from the results of Fisher et al. documenting that preoperative timing of only the low but not the high dose of cyclophosphamide was superior when compared with its postoperative introduction in mice mammary systems (Fisher et al. 1983). Preoperative chemotherapy is not consistently superior - van Putten's experiments showed its advantage in mice mammary but not in the lung tumor models (Mulder et al. 1983).

Despite occasional opinions to the contrary, many clinical investigators have accepted the presently available theoretical and experimental evidence and the rationale for preoperative chemotherapy as sufficiently convincing to consider its testing in human tumors. The data of such therapy for osteogenic sarcoma (Rosen 1982), head and neck (Schuller 1983), and locally advanced breast cancer tumors (Schick et al. 1983; Aisner and Morris 1982; Perloff and Lesnick 1982) attest to the possibility that, in addition to its expected advantage for overall survival, other benefits can be expected. Preoperative chemotherapy may enable an in vivo assessment of its effectiveness, enabling clinicians a more scientific approach toward the selection of individual patients and chemotherapy agents for adjuvant therapy of cancer. As well, preoperative chemotherapy may allow a more uniform adoption of conservative surgery as seen from the preliminary data on osteogenic sarcoma (Rosen 1982) and breast cancer (Jacquillat et al. 1983). Of further value for the locoregional disease are data documenting that previously inoperable disease may be rendered operable (Perloff and Lesnick 1982; Sokolova 1980). Thus, a palliative treatment may be converted into a curative approach.

The British Columbia Trial of Neoadjuvant Therapy of Breast Cancer

Preoperative chemotherapy for stage I and II breast cancer started in our region in 1981. In the first phase of the project, a pilot study of 43 patients was completed and presented on several occasions (Ragaz et al. 1983; 1984). Subsequently, randomization of the premenopausal patients with established diagnosis of breast cancer in the preoperative and postoperative arms was started (Table 3) with 68 patients enrolled in the study until February 1985. The preliminary analysis of the study will be briefly outlined.

The Role of Fine-Needle Aspiration in the Diagnosis of Breast Cancer

Part of our phase 1 study of the neoadjuvant therapy of breast cancer included introduction, in our region, of fine-needle aspiration (FNA) as a primary method to establish a diagnosis of breast cancer. Its advantages over the conventionally performed two-stage incisional biopsy are multiple and were discussed in more detail in our previous reports

(Ragaz et al. 1983; 1984) as well as in the literature (Zajicek 1974; Frable 1983). A review of the published material shows that in centers with an experienced cytologist, and a suspicious mammogram and clinical examination, the accuracy of FNA can be very high, with diagnostic error decreased to 1%. Despite its popularity in many European institutions, FNA as the only diagnostic method is presently only infrequently performed in North America. Further attempts to popularize this technique in Canada and the United States will be needed.

Pilot Study of Neoadjuvant Chemotherapy

In the pilot study, one course of preoperative chemotherapy with CMF was given to 43 patients with newly diagnosed breast cancer. We concluded that such treatment was safe, as there had been no case of mortality and it was shown that wound healing and other morbidity had not substantially differed from the patients undergoing mastectomy without preoperative chemotherapy (Ragaz et al. 1983; 1984). As well, gastrointestinal

Table 2. Regimen of the British Columbia randomized trial of preoperative versus postoperative adjuvant chemotherapy for premenopausal patients with newly diagnosed carcinoma of the breast (70)[a]

Regimen	
1	Preoperative CMF[b] × 1 Surgery Postoperative CMF × 8
2	Surgery Postoperative CMF × 9

[a] For both arms: chest wall XRT after the fourth cycle of CMF
[b] *CMF*, cyclophosphamide 600 mg/m^2 i.v., methotrexate 50 mg/m^2 i.v., 5-fluorouracil 600 mg/m^2 i.v. The CMF regimen is given every 3 weeks

Table 3. British Columbia randomized trial of preoperative versus postoperative adjuvant chemotherapy for premenopausal patients with cancer of the breast - nodal status and tumor

Site		Preoperative (34)[a] (%)	Postoperative (34)[a] (%)
	0	54	58
Nodes	1-3	31	31
	3-7	17	10
Tumor	2	54	61
Size (cm)	2-5	37	30
	>5	8	9

[a] Number of patients in each group

Table 4. Delay between the diagnosis and the first cycle of chemotherapy (DG-CT-INT) versus the allocated randomized group. Postoperative (post) adjuvant chemotherapy of breast cancer, British Columbia trial

	Preoperative (34)[a]	Postoperative (18)[a]	*P*
DG-CT-INT (days)	6	24	< 0.0001
SD		16	

[a] Number of patients analyzed

and bone marrow toxicities in patients from the pilot study were similar to those seen in the 420 patients at our institution receiving the same adjuvant chemotherapy in the conventional postoperative setting.

Randomized study of Neoadjuvant Therapy

In 1983, randomization of the premenopausal patients with newly diagnosed breast cancer into the preoperative and postoperative treatment groups was started. As of February 1985, 68 patients were randomized, with 34 patients allocated into each arm. As a result of the more frequent ongoing introductory sessions with the community surgeons, 16 unfunded private practitioners contributed patients to the randomized study, whereas only 2 surgeons did so to the pilot study. Presently, the randomization is done by the surgeon after the tissue diagnosis of breast cancer has been obtained. After the randomization is obtained, those patients randomized to the preoperative arm will have the first course of preoperative chemotherapy given, soon after the investigations are ordered. The date of the definitive surgery is presently not altered and is similar to its timing in patients randomized to the postoperative arm or to patients not participating in the preoperative study. The surgery, for patients randomized in both arms, is either modified radical mastectomy (42 patients) or partial mastectomy (26 patients). The latter operation consists of the resection of the quadrant containing the tumor and of axillary sampling done through a separate axillary incision. After the surgery, the high-risk patients from both groups receive postoperative chemotherapy consisting of eight (for patients from the preoperative arm) or nine (for patients from the postoperative arm) CMF cycles given every 3 weeks (Table 2). The high-risk features determining the need for postoperative chemotherapy consist of either positive axiallary lymph glands or in the case of negative axillary lymph glands, of histological evidence of vascular or lymphangitic spread in the primary tumor. The patients with negative axillary lymph nodes and low-risk features receive no postoperative chemotherapy. Chest wall radiotherapy (3750 R in 15 fractions) follows the fourth cycle of CMF chemotherapy and is given to all patients with positive axillary lymph nodes, to those axillary node-negative patients whose tumors are located in the medial and central quadrants, and to those women who have undergone partial mastectomy (lumpectomy). After the radiotherapy, chemotherapy treatments continue for five more cycles. Table 3 shows the outline of the nodal status and tumor size, indicating their even distribution in both randomized groups. Of interest is the fact that over 50% patients from both groups had negative axillary lymph and tumors less than 2 cm in size. All of the axillary node-negative patients randomized to the preoperative chemotherapy arm received

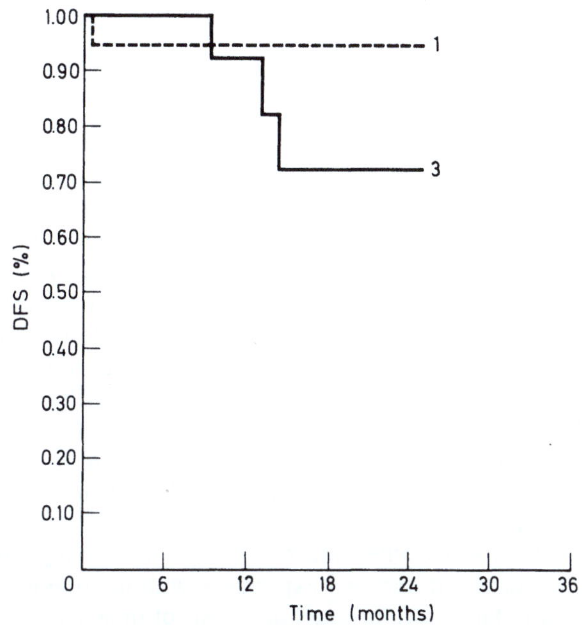

Fig. 2. British Columbia randomized study of preoperative (34 patients) versus postoperative (34 patients) adjuvant chemotherapy for premenopausal patients with breast cancer; disease-free survival *(DFS)* at two years follow up shows no significant difference; ($P = > 0.1$). Figures in parentheses = number of failures

one or more cycles of CMF, whereas only 24% of the patients of the same category, randomized to the postoperative chemotherapy arm, received chemotherapy treatment ($P = < 0.0001$).

Estrogen receptor assay showed similar distribution in both randomized arms, with the mean ER (estrogen receptor) value of 36 and 24 fmol/mg cytosol protein in both groups respectively ($P = > 0.5$). The interval between the diagnosis and the first cycle of chemotherapy was 6 and 24 days respectively ($P = < 0.0001$) (Table 4). The disease-free survival at 2 years follow-up shows no statistically significant difference ($P = > 0.1$) between the randomized arms (Fig. 2).

Future Aspects of Neoadjuvant Treatment of Breast Cancer: Discussion

Despite the convincing theoretical and experimental data indicating superiority of preoperative over postoperative adjuvant chemotherapy, preoperative chemotherapy has not yet been sufficiently tested in human malignancies. If adopted on a large scale, the treatment with preoperative chemotherapy will alter the present management of breast cancer and many details of the conventional and traditional approaches toward the diagnosis, staging, and therapy will change significantly. Therefore, before the preoperative chemotherapy can be recommended as a standard treatment, a thorough analysis of its rationale and cost benefit will have to be available.

In this paper, a short review of the main biological phenomena of cancer in connection with the preoperative chemotherapy is presented, indicating its theoretical advantage over the postoperative chemotherapy. The data of our pilot study show that the treatment of newly diagnosed premenopausal breast cancer patients with one cycle of CMF was well tolerated. The preliminary analysis of our randomized study of preoperative versus postoperative adjuvant chemotherapy for the same population of patients is described, further confirming the safety and no undue side effects of the preoperative treatment. Other aspects of the neoadjuvant approach include the fine-needle aspiration for the initial diagnosis of breast cancer. Involvement of unfunded private practitioners, in particular of surgeons, is felt to be of primary importance. Without their continuous support with both the randomization as well as with the organization of the preoperative treatment, the neoadjuvant trials cannot continue. It is presently felt that their willingness in our region to participate is the single most important factor determining the viability of the present project. Continuous upgrading and education of the various communities of surgeons throughout British Columbia is presently done regularly by the principal investigators. It remains to be shown whether such an approach without a financial renumeration of the practitionsers will remain a stimulus effective enough to maintain their continuous interest in the randomization and eventually in the future, in the routine practice of preoperative chemotherapy.

What about other future aspects of the neoadjuvant treatment? From the review of the literature and our own experience with the fine-needle aspiration as the only diagnostic method to obtain primary diagnosis of breat cancer, it is felt that the presently performed open biopsy may likely be replaced by this technique, permitting a faster and more efficient organization of the first phase of breast cancer management. Its potential benefits with regard to tumor kinetics over the open biopsy have been discussed, making us to believe that FNA may soon be practiced by more centers. Other new developments linked to the preoperative chemotherapy are likely to take place. One has to consider a possibility that effective intensive preoperative chemotherapy treatments may sterilize a proportion of positive axillary lymph glands, rendering the presently performed pathological staging uninterpretable. Hence, information on the prechemotherapy assessment will be needed to define the high-risk patients. The neoadjuvant staging, in addition to the clinical TNM assessment, will likely utilize information from the history (Boyd et al. 1981), serial mammography examinations (Heuser et al. 1979), and flow cytometry (Auer and Tribukait 1980; Kute et al. 1981). This latter technique, examining tissue obtained by either FNA or open biopsy, allows an accurate assessment of tumor DNA content, ploidy, as well as cellular differentiation. These indices, as shown in the preliminary reviews (Fisher et al. 1983; Olszewski et al. 1981; Jakesz et al. 1985), correlate well with subsequent prognosis, both with the recurrence rate as well as with the overall survival. In addition, information on estrogen receptors (Olszeski et al. 1981) and on serial chemotherapy uptake by the tumor (Durand and Olive 1981) as obtained from flow cytometry, could be effectively utilized in daily practice, enlarging thus the scope of neoadjuvant staging. The neoadjuvant approach may, therefore, permit a more scientific approach, allowing, in addition to other advantages, a maximum selectivity in the choice of therapeutic options for individualized subgroups of patients according to their risk category.

In summary, evidence is presented which indicates that preoperative timing of adjuvant chemotherapy and other aspects of the neoadjuvant approach may further improve the results of the conventional adjuvant therapies. Presently, however, despite its logical and scientific rationale, insufficient clinical evidence of its true advantage over the postoperative approach is available. Therefore, despite its relative safety as documented in our study, further trials of preoperative adjuvant chemotherapy in breast cancer are indicated.

References

Aisner J, Mooris D (1982) Mastectomy as an adjuvant to chemotherapy for locally advanced or metastatic cancer. Arch Surg 17: 882-887

Auer G, Tribukait B (1980) Comparative single cell and flow DNA analysis in aspiration biopsies from breast carcinomas. Acta Pathol Microbiol Scand 88 A: 355-358

Boyd NF, Meakin JW, Hayward JL, et al (1981) Clinical estimation of the growth rate of breast cancer. Cancer 48: 1037-1042

Buzdar AU, Smith TL, Powell KC, et al (1982) Effect of timing of initiation of adjuvant chemotherapy of disease free survival in breast cancer. Breast Cancer Res Treat 2: 163-169

Corbett TH, Griswold DP Jr, Roberts BJ, et al (1978) Biology and therapeutic response of a mouse mammary adenocarcinoma (16/C) and its potential as a model for surgical adjuvant chemotherapy. Cancer Treat Rep 62: 1471-1488

DeWyss WD (1972) Studies correlating the growth rate of tumor and its metastases providing evidence for tumor related systemic growth retarding factors. Cancer Res 32: 374-379

Durand RE, Olive PL (1981) Flow cytometry studies of intracellular Adriamycin in single cells in vitro. Cancer Res 41: 3489-3494

Fisher B, Gunduz N, Saffer EA (1983) Influence of the interval between primary tumor removal and chemotherapy on kinetics and growth of metastases. Cancer Res 43: 1488-1492

Frable WJ (1983) Fine needle aspiration biopsy: a review. Hum Pathol 14: 9-28

Glucksberg H, Rivkin SE, Rasmussen S, et al (1982) Combination chemotherapy (DMFVP) versus L-phenylalanine mustard (L-PAM) for operable breast cancer with positive axillary nodes. Cancer 50: 423-434

Goldhirsch A (1983) Toxic effects of early adjuvant chemotherapy for breast cancer. Lancet 2: 542-544

Goldie JH, Coldman AJ (1979) A mathematical model for relating the drug sensitivity of tumors to their spontaneous mutation rate. Cancer Treat Rep 63: 1727-1733

Gorelik E, Segal S, Feldman M (1978) Growth of a local tumor exerts a specific inhibitory effect on progression of lung metastases. Int J Cancer 21: 617-625

Heuser L, Spratt JS, Polk HC Jr (1979) Growth rates of primary breast cancers. Cancer 43: 1888-1894

Jacquillat C, Baillet F, Blondon J, et al (1983) Preliminary results of "neoadjuvant" chemotherapy in initial management of breast cancer (BC). Proc Am Soc Clin Oncol 2: C-437, 112

Jakesz R, Kolb R, Reiner G et al (1985) Effect of adjuvant chemotherapy in Stages I and II breast cancer is dependent on tumor differentiation and estrogen receptor status. Am Soc Clin Oncol 4: C-265, 69

Jones SE, Brooks RJ, Takasugi BJ, et al (1984) Current results of the University of Arizona adjuvant breast cancer trials (1974-1984). In: Senn SJ (ed) Adjuvant chemotherapy of breast cancer. Springer, Berlin Heidelberg New York Tokyo, pp 133-141 (Recent results in cancer research, vol 96)

Kute TE, Muss HB, Anderson D, et al (1981) Relationship of steroid receptor, cell kinetics and clinical status in patients with breast cancer. Cancer Res 41: 3524-3529

Mulder JH, deRuiter JD, Edelstein MB, Gerritsen TFC, van Putten LM (1983) Model studies in adjuvant chemotherapy. Cancer Treat Rep 67: 45-50

Nissen-Meyer R, Kjellgren K, Malmio K et al (1978) Surgical adjuvant chemotherapy: results with one short course with cyclophosphamide after mastectomy for breast cancer. Cancer 41: 2088-2098

Olszewski W, Darzynkiewicz Z, Rosen PP, et al (1981) Flow cytometry of breast carcinoma: relation of DNA ploidy level to histology and estrogen receptor. Cancer 48: 980-984

Perloff M, Lesnick J (1982) Chemotherapy before and after mastectomy in Stage III breast cancer. Arch Surg 117: 879-881

Ragaz J, Baird R, Goldie J, et al (1983) Neoadjuvant - preoperative (preop) adjuvant chemotherapy (CT) for breast cancer - new approach for the management of breast cancer. Proc Am Soc Clin Oncol 2: C-434, 111

Ragaz J, Baird R, Goldie J, Rebbeck P, Spinelli J (1984) Neoadjuvant (preoperative) chemotherapy for breast cancer. In: Salmon SE, Jones SE (eds) Adjuvant therapy of cancer IV. Grune and Stratton, Orlando, pp 425-433

Ragaz J, Baird R, Rebbeck P, et al (1985) Neoadjuvant (preoperative) chemotherapy for breast cancer. Cancer 56: 719-725

Rosen G (1982) Preoperative chemotherapy for osteogenic sarcoma. Cancer 49: 1221-1230

Schick P, Goodstein J, Moor J, et al (1983) Preoperative chemotherapy followed by mastectomy for locally advanced breast cancer. J Surg Oncol 22: 278-282

Schuller DE (1983) Preoperative reductive chemotherapy for locally advanced carcinoma of the oral cavity, oropharynx, and hypopharynx. Cancer 51: 15-19

Senn HJ, Jungi WF, Amgwerd R (1981) Chemo(immuno)therapy with LFMP plus BCG in node negative and node positve breast cancer. In: Salmon SE, Jones SE (eds) Adjuvant therapy of cancer III. Grune and Stratton, San Francisco, pp 385-395

Simpson-Herren L, Sanford AH, Holmquist JP (1976) Effects of surgery on the cell kinetics of residual tumor. Cancer Treat Rep 60: 1749-1760

Sokolova IG (1980) Preoperative poly chemotherapy in the complex treatment of locally spread cancer of the mammary gland. Vopr Onkol 26: 9-13

Zajicek J (1974) Aspiration biopsy cytology: I. Cytology of supradiaphragmatic organs. In: Karger, New York

Perioperative Adjuvant Chemotherapy of Breast Cancer: The Scandinavian Experience

R. Nissen-Meyer, H. Host, K. Kjellgren, B. Mansson, and T. Norin*

Tyribakken 10, 0280 Oslo 2, Norway

Introduction

In several clinical trials it has been shown that adjuvant chemotherapy may reduce the number of recurrences after a mastectomy for breast cancer, or significantly delay their clinical appearance.

An overview at a meeting held in London on 24-26 October 1984 of the mortality data from all such available trials (including over 10000 women) revealed a significant ($P <$ 0.001) reduction in short-term mortality in the groups with long-term adjuvant chemotherapy (UK Breast Cancer Trials Coordinating Subcommittee and Project on Controlled Therapeutic Trials of the UICC 1984).

On the other hand, it has become increasingly clear that side effects from long-term chemotherapy may seriously impair the quality of life after mastectomy.

The Scandinavian Adjuvant Chemotherapy Study Group since 1965 has tested a single, short perioperative adjuvant chemotherapy course which has virtually negligible side effects, and since 1977 has compared such a course with a cyclophosphamide, methotrexate, and 5-fluorouracil (CMF) schedule for 12 months.

Material and Methods

The case material was primary breast cancer patients, considered fit for mastectomy according to the routine procedures of the local hospitals.

The design of our two studies is summarized in Fig. 1.

Study 1 started in January 1965; the intake was closed in September 1975. One-half of the patients were randomized before 30 July 1969.

The main subseries included 1026 patients. They were randomized by telephone from the operating theatre, and in the treatment group (507 cases) chemotherapy started after closure of the surgical wound. The chemotherapy group received cyclophosphamide i.v. 5 mg/kg per day for 6 days. Both groups had postoperative radiotherapy. The delay between mastectomy and start of radiotherapy (in some hospitals only 4 days) was not influenced by the chemotherapy given.

The smaller subseries (110 cases) consisted of patients from the Radiotherapy Institute of the University of Helsinki. They arrived at the Institute between 2 and 4 weeks after a

* The members of the Scandinavian Adjuvant Chemotherapy Study Group are listed in Appendix A

Recent Results in Cancer Research. Vol 103

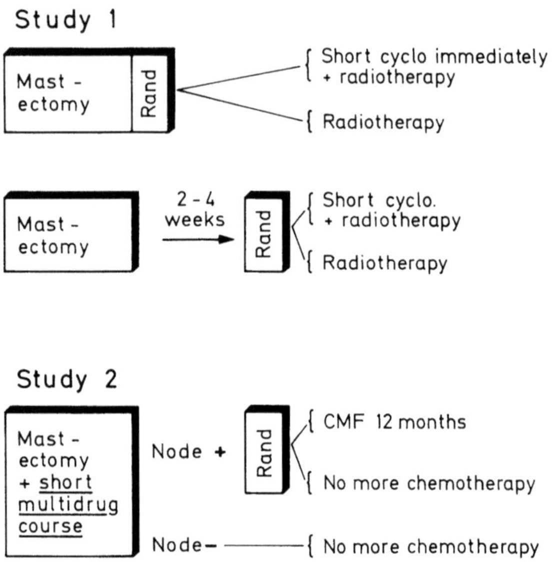

Fig. 1. Study design

mastectomy performed in other hospitals, and were randomized after arrival, on average 21 days after mastectomy. From then on the procedure was the same as in the larger sub-series.

The only stratification before randomization in study 1 was by hospital.

Study 2 started in March 1977; the study is still open.

All patients now receive one short chemotherapy course immediately after mastectomy. In light of the general development in cancer chemotherapy between 1965 and 1977, we changed our monodrug course to a multidrug course with cyclophosphamide 500 mg, vincristine 1 mg, and 5-fluorouracil (5-FU) 750 mg on day 0 and cyclophosphamide 500 mg, vincristine 1 mg, and methotrexate 50 mg on day 7; i. v. All doses stated are for a patient of 70 kg or more, and were adjusted for lower weights.

After stratification, the 367 axillary-node-positive patients were randomly allotted to an experimental group advised to continue with CMF for 1 year or to a control group with no further adjuvant chemotherapy other than the perioperative course already given. The patients allotted to the experimental group were strongly encouraged to take and continue the CMF treatment, but were told that it was a clinical trial, and that they might stop the treatment at any time if they found the side effects intolerable. They were informed that such treatment was routine in many major centers in the world.

Doses for the long-term CMF treatment were cyclophosphamide 500 mg, methotrexate 50 mg, and 5-FU 750 mg i. v. on day 1 and 8 in each 4-week cycle, for 12 cycles (doses for a patient of 70 kg).

The 737 axillary-node-negative patients received no further adjuvant chemotherapy.

Treatment after diagnosis of relapse was left to the discretion of the local hospital, in both studies.

(One-half of the patients in study 2 were also randomized to receive immunotherapy with *Corynebacterium parvum* given subcutaneously around the mastectomy scar. This treatment has shown no effect on the overall results so far and will be ignored in this presentation. The immunotherapy part of our study will be reported on a later occasion.)

Beneficial Effects

Figure 2 shows the relapse-free percentages and the crude survival percentages in the main subseries of study 2, as they were found in March 1976, March 1978, March 1980, and at the latest follow-up, in September 1984.

In 1976, the difference between the relapse-free rates was small during the first few years after mastectomy, but increased thereafter, demonstrating a benefit for the group with the immediate, short cyclophosphamide course, significant at $P < 0.001$. Until 1984 this pattern was kept unchanged, with a follow-up of 18 years. Both curves seem to have reached a plateau.

The crude survival rates also showed a significant benefit for the treatment group in 1976 ($P < 0.01$). The difference appeared later than the difference in relapse rates, but increased and was maintained for the entire follow-up time of 10 years. During the following years, however, the crude survival curves did not reach a plateau. They both continued to decline, the difference between them was reduced, and in 1984 the formal significance had disappeared.

The case material of study 1 had a relatively high age at entry. The mean age was 55.5, the median 55.06, the range 27-84 years. Our eligibility criteria had stated an upper age of 70 years, but our committee decided not to exclude the few patients randomized above that age. There was no difference between the two treatment groups, with a mean age of 55.4 and 55.6 years respectively.

Between March 1976 and September 1984 the median age of the case material increased from 61.7 to 70.3 years.

Figure 3 shows a comparison between the results obtained in the two subseries of study 1, evaluated as relapse-free survival. The only difference between the treatment given in these two subseries was that in the larger one the short chemotherapy course was giv-

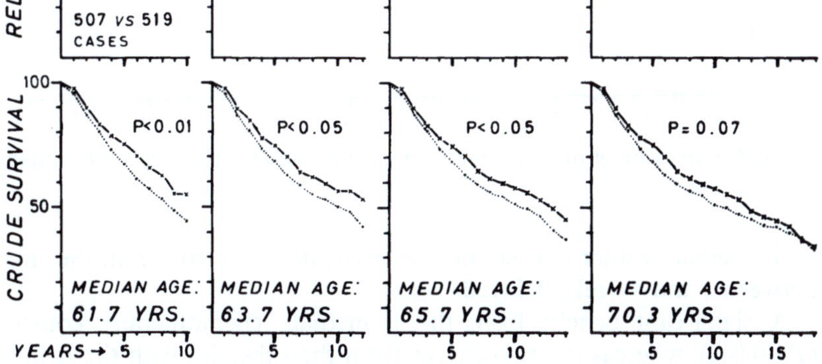

Fig. 2. Effect of the short perioperative cyclophosphamide course as observed in 1976, 1978, 1980, and 1984

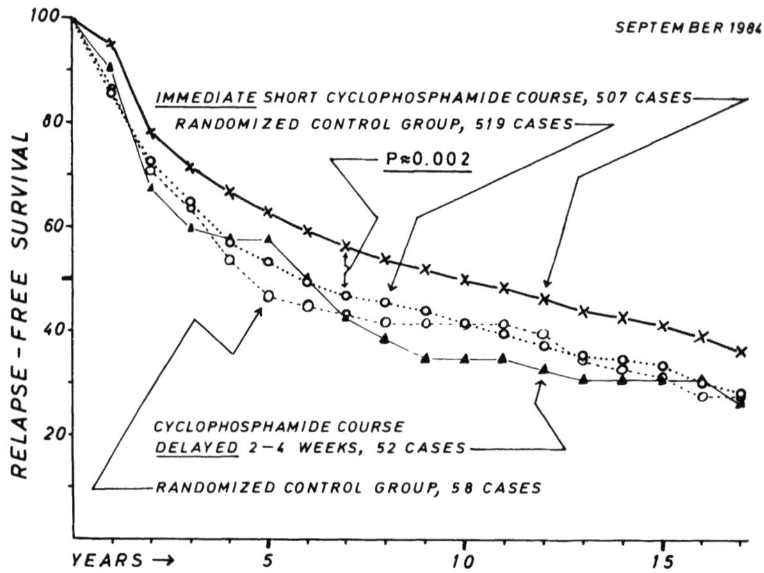

Fig. 3. Comparison of the perioperative and the delayed short cyclophosphamide courses

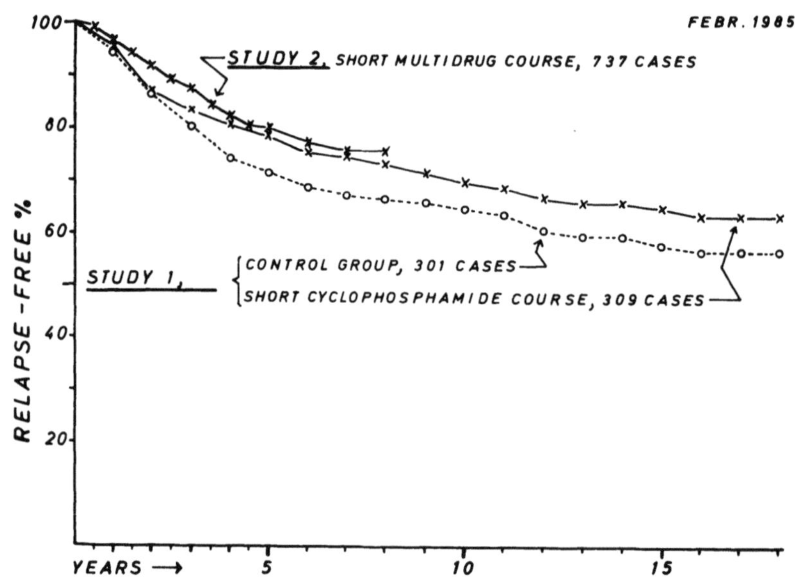

Fig. 4. Comparison of the short multidrug course and the short cyclophosphamide course in node-negative cases

en immediately after mastectomy, whereas the same course in the smaller subseries was between 2 and 4 weeks delayed.

A significant benefit from the immediate chemotherapy course is demonstrated ($P \sim 0.002$), whereas the two curves from the subseries with the delayed course demonstrate no trend of an effect. They are statistically indistinguishable from the control curve of the subseries with the immediate course.

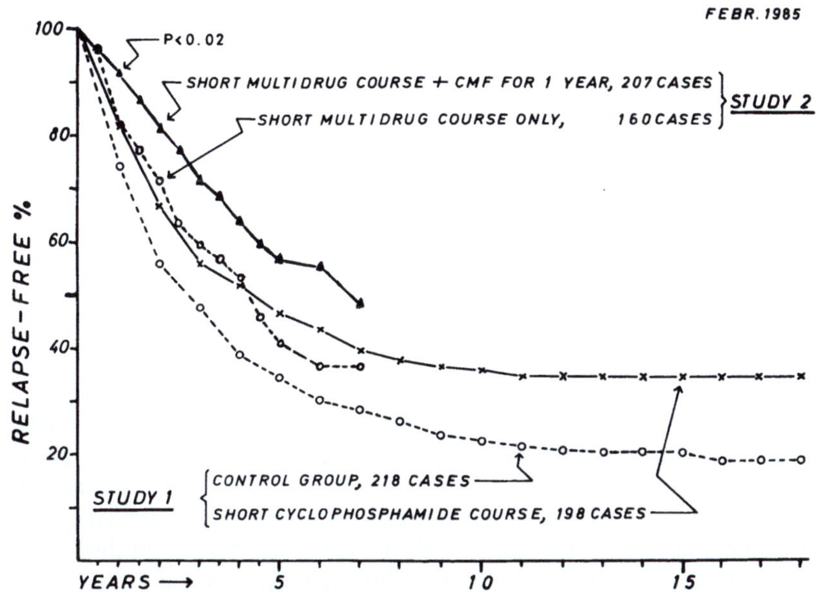

Fig. 5. Comparison of the prolonged CMF treatment and the single, short courses in node-positive cases

Figure 4 compares the relapse-free rates in the node-negative cases from both studies. After 18 years the difference between the two groups of study 1 is 7%, suggesting that with the short cyclophosphamide course 16% of the 44% relapses seen in the control group had been avoided with the single, short course.

The result in the 737 cases of study 2 is slightly better than the result in the cyclophosphamide group of study 1, suggesting that the multidrug course used is at least as effective as the cyclophosphamide course was.

Figure 5 compares the relapse-free rates in the node-positive cases from both studies. After 18 years the difference between the two groups of study 1 is 16%, suggesting that with the short cyclophosphamide course 19.5% of the 81.5% relapses seen in the control group had been avoided with the single, short course.

The result in the control group of study 2 is indistinguishable from the result of the experimental group of study 1, suggesting that the multidrug course is as effective as the cyclophosphamide course.

The result in the new experimental group (207 cases) with CMF for 1 year is significantly better than the results in the two groups with only one single perioperative course ($P < 0.02$). This difference is diminishing after some years.

Side Effects

The immediate side effects of the single perioperative courses were of short duration and virtually negligible. They mainly consisted of some nausea which was easy to palliate, since the patients were still in hospital after mastectomy. The short bone marrow suppression caused no problem, and the treatment did not interfere with a normal healing of the surgical wound (Nissen-Meyer et al. 1978).

Table 1. Second malignancies observed in study 1 (excluding breast cancer and basocellular skin cancer)

	Short cyclophosphamide group	Control group
Leukemia and lymphoma	2	4
Gynecological cancer	3	6
Gastrointestinal cancer	8	7
Other neoplasms	5	6
Total	18	23

There is no indication that the single cyclophosphamide course has induced second neoplasms. With 1136 patients randomized and up to 19 years of follow-up we have observed 41 cases of leukemia, lymphomas, and secondary carcinomas (Table 1), 23 in the control group and 18 in the treated group. What we have observed is the general tendency of patients surviving one cancer to develop another malignant disease.

It is still too early to evaluate second malignancies in study 2.

The long-term CMF treatment, however, represented a serious problem. Only 36% of the patients managed to complete this treatment with at least 90% of the scheduled dose. The side effects were considered mild in 23%, moderate in 29%, and severe in 48% of those who completed the treatment.

For the remaining patients the dose had to be reduced due to the side effects; 37% received between 50% and 90% of the scheduled dose, 21% less than 50% of this total dose. Only 5% of the patients refused to start with the CMF treatment they were offered.

Nausea and vomiting tended to increase in severity with increasing number of courses, and could continue for a whole week after each injection.

A reduction of the doses usually had little effect on this pattern of side effects, when it was first established.

As a consequence, 41% of the patients who started with CMF eventually insisted that the treatment should be terminated, and they did so after a median of 6½ courses (13 injections).

The first three to four courses were usually fairly well tolerated, but after this most of the patients felt the continued treatment as a heavy burden.

Discussion

Relapse-Free Percentage, Crude Survival, or Relapse-Free Survival as a Measure of Adjuvant Chemotherapy Effect?

Figure 2 may serve as an example for this discussion.

Relapse-free percentage is specific, counting as an "event" only demonstrating relapses of the specific cancer, whereas patients dying from other causes without a demonstrated relapse are censored as observed only until the time of death.

However, the method includes some subjective judgments, for instance, if there is or is not a reason to suspect that the death had been due to cancer, even if this was not recorded on the death certificate, and judgment about the time the relapse should have first been registered.

On the other hand, crude survival is objective. The only "event" that is counted is death – there may be no discussion if a patient is dead or alive, and the time of death is an exact date. The effect of the treatment is of course seen later in crude survival rates than in relapse rates.

However, crude survival is an unspecific method for assessing the effect of a cancer treatment. The older the case material is, and the longer the observation time, the more unspecific deaths will be observed, deaths unrelated to the original disease and not influenced by the treatment studied. Eventually, all patients will have died in both treatment groups and the difference in crude survival rates between the groups will accordingly be zero.

Crude survival rates are also influenced by secondary treatment after diagnosis of the first recurrence. This secondary treatment does not influence the relapse-free percentage.

However, even if in some instances the relapse-free % may be seen as the most appropriate method for assessing the response, crude survival should also be computed at the same time, to control possible unforeseen side effects of the treatment which might influence survival.

Relapse-free survival counts both recurrences and death as an "event," whichever of these two events comes first. It has both the advantages and the disadvantages of the two other methods.

There can be no doubt about the effect of the short perioperative cyclophosphamide course, measured as relapse-free rates. The difference was maintained for at least 18 years after mastectomy. The curves seem to have reached a plateau, which means that possible uncertainties about the right time to register a relapse have lost their importance.

The specific effect seen in the relapse-free percentages is objectively confirmed by the significant difference in crude survival rates found some years ago. After this more and more deaths unrelated to breast cancer have blurred the picture, and the formal significance is now lost. This, however, does not reduce the significance of the benefit in crude survival rates found in 1976. In September 1984 one-half of the patients were, or would have been, more than 70 years old. Only 34% of the patients were alive 18 years after mastectomy, whereas in 46% a recurrence had never been found.

The consequence is that with a really long follow-up time in case material with a relatively high age, we must rely more on relapse rates and less on crude survival rates, if we want a specific picture of the effect of a primary treatment method. This is even more important when we want to compare results obtained in various randomized series with different age distributions.

Evaluation of the Short Perioperative Course. With one single, short perioperative course we have observed a highly significant benefit in relapse-free rates, and also a significant crude survival benefit. These results get some support from the late observations of the early trial of the NSABP with one short perioperative course with thiotepa (Fisher et al. 1968). In our study the effect seems to be the same in node-negative and node-positive, in pre- and postmenopausal patients (Nissen-Meyer et al. 1982).

The pattern of effect cannot be explained only by a delaying influence on the course of the disease; the effect observed must be due to a true increase in cure rate.

The cost of this adjuvant treatment in terms of side effects has been almost negligible, but also the financial cost is very modest. Cyclophosphamide is very cheap, and the resources necessary to administer it are small. In fact, every hospital in the world, capable of performing a decent mastectomy, will also be able to give this type of adjuvant chemotherapy.

Evaluation of the Prolonged Adjuvant Chemotherapy. Prolongation of chemotherapy to 1 year has shown a significant benefit in relapse-free rates. It seems, however, that the effect is diminishing after some years, indicating that the extra benefit obtained may at least partly be an extra delay of the disease, instead of an increased cure rate. In a few years time we may have more reliable information on this point.

On the other hand, the extra benefit of prolonging chemotherapy to 1 year - whatever this benefit may be shown to be - has been obtained at a rather high cost in terms of side effects and reduced "quality of life." Also expenses and the necessary resources are considerably increased, and may under certain circumstances be inhibitory.

The induced, and increasing, aversion against cytotoxic drugs must necessarily have a negative influence upon the chance for a succesful treatment of a recurrent disease later.

However, the first three to four courses of prolonged chemotherapy were usually much better tolerated than the later courses. A reduction from the duration of 12 months to 4 months would considerably improve the "quality of life" after mastectomy, and at the same time reduce the cost and the resources needed. A new trial, with a long follow-up time, comparing the benefit of treatment for 4 versus 12 months with chemotherapy starting immediately after mastectomy, is needed.

Appendix A. Members of the Scandinavian Adjuvant Chemotherapy Study Group

Finland
Helsinki: A. A. Järvinen†, L. Holsti, K. Malmio†; Oulu: G. Blanco, T. Larmi, Vasa: P. O. Grönblom

Norway
Akershus: I. Broyn, N. Helsingen, E. W. Vaagenes; Bergen: T. Kolsaker, B. Rosengren, M. Tangen, J. E. Varhaug; Bodo: R. Aune, R. Capoferro, S. M. Sivertsen; Lillehammer: I. Hareide, S. K. Hjort; Oslo: I. O. Brennhovd, S. Gundersen, S. Hagen, T. Harbitz, H. Host, O. G. Jorgensen, S. Kvaløy, H. O. Myhre, R. Nissen-Meyer (coordinator)

Sweden
Boras: S. Ahlström, C.-A. Ekman, B. Månsson; Gavle: G. Hellström, T. Norin, G. Odén; Jönkoping: I. Iacobaeus, B. Mårtensson; Kalmar: B. Pallin; Linköping: J. Saaf, D. Turesson; Norrköping: H. O. Ahnlund, K. Kjellgren, R. Peterhoff; Vastervik: K. Wiegner

References

Fisher B, Ravdin RG, Ausman RK, Slack NH, Moore GE, Noer RJ (1968) Surgical adjuvant chemotherapy in cancer of the breast; results of a decade of cooperative investigation. Ann Surg 168: 337-356

Nissen-Meyer R, Kjellgren K, Malmio K, Mansson B, Norin T (1978) Surgical adjuvant chemotherapy. Results with one short course with cyclophosphamide after mastectomy for breast cancer. Cancer 41: 2088-2098

Nissen-Meyer R, Kjellgren K, Mansson B (1982) Adjuvant chemotherapy in breast cancer. Springer, Berlin Heidelberg New York, pp 142-148 (Recent results in cancer research, vol 80)

UK Breast Cancer Trials Coordinating Subcommittee and Project on Controlled Therapeutic Trials of the UICC (1984) Review of mortality results in randomized trials in early breast cancer. Lancet ii: 1205

Perioperative and Conventionally Timed Chemotherapy in Operable Breast Cancer: The Ludwig Breast Cancer Study V

A. Goldhirsch and R. Gelber*

Ludwig Institute for Cancer Research, Inselspital, 3010 Bern, Switzerland

Adjuvant systemic therapy in operable breast cancer has been shown to produce a disease-free survival advantage and a reduction in mortality (Bonadonna et al. 1978; Joint BCTC/WHO/UICC Overview 1984). It has been suggested that treatment success may well be dose related (Bonadonna and Valagussa 1981; Bonadonna et al. 1981) and toxicity related (Carpenter et al. 1982).

A number of strategies have been proposed in recent years to improve the results of current adjuvant therapy. These include:

1. The use of non-cross-resistant drug combinations
2. More intensive and prolonged use of existing drugs
3. Combination of chemo- and hormone therapies and/or immunotherapy (Hubay et al. 1981)
4. The use of investigational drugs
5. Early commencement of chemotherapy after surgery

Sequential use of non-cross-resistant drugs and more intensive chemotherapy are being evaluated by other groups. The current investigational drugs seem unlikely to be better than existing agents in the adjuvant setting. The Ludwig Breast Cancer Studies I-IV explored chemohormonotherapy combinations between 1978 and 1981. Additional follow-up is warranted so that significant data from these trials can be made available.

The time of starting chemotherapy after removal of the primary tumor may be of critical based on experimental, kinetic, and drug resistance considerations (Goldie and Coldman 1979; Schabel 1977; Dewys 1972; Fisher et al. 1983) and on certain clinical evidence (Fisher et al. 1975; Nissen-Meyer et al. 1978). Two clinical trials which started chemotherapy in the immediate postoperative period showed survival advantages in at least some of the patient subpopulations. The NSABP study using perioperative thiotepa revealed a significant survival advantage in premenopausal patients with four or more nodes involved (Fisher et al. 1975). The Scandinavian Adjuvant Chemotherapy Study Group used cyclophosphamide for 6 days from the day of mastectomy and demonstrated a survival advantage of about 15% overall after more than 15 years (Nissen-Meyer et al., this volume). This benefit applied almost equally to N+ and N−, pre- and postmenopausal patients, and was lost when adjuvant chemotherapy was delayed by as little as 3 weeks. It therefore seems logical, even essential, to evaluate the effects of starting chemotherapy immediately following surgery rather than to expose the patient to the possible deleterious effects of delay.

---

* The participants of the Ludwig Cancer Study Group are listed on p. 110, 111

Study Design

In order to study this aspect of timing in the adjuvant treatment of breast cancer the Ludwig Breast Cancer Study Group initiated a trial (LBCS V) using perioperative treatment administered in the immediately postoperative phase. The study design is shown in Fig. 1.

Two-thirds of the node-negative patients receive perioperative chemotherapy only, while one-third receive no further therapy after the mastectomy. Of the N+ patients, one-third receive only conventionally timed chemotherapy, starting within 25–36 days after mastectomy, one-third receive only the perioperative chemotherapy, and one-third receive perioperative chemotherapy followed by conventionally timed chemotherapy. The trial was begun in November 1981, after a pilot study of 65 patients treated with the perioperative regimen indicated that tolerance was acceptable.

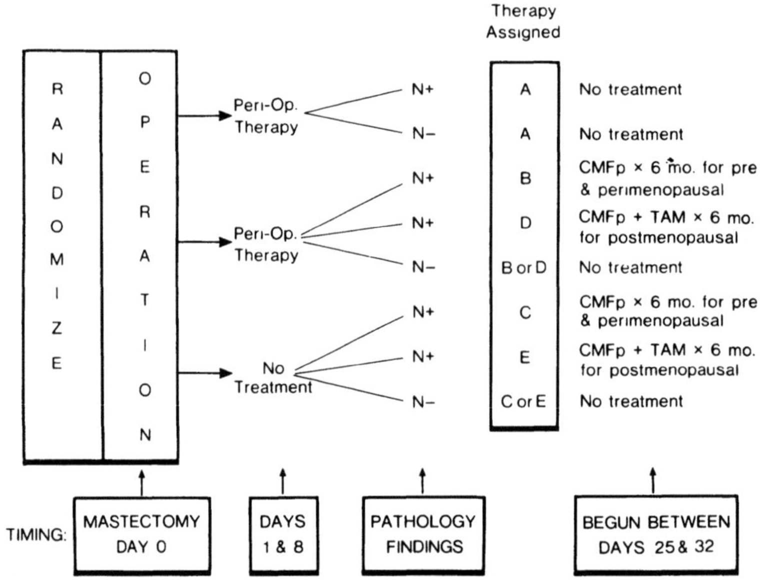

Fig. 1. Schema of the Ludwig Breast Cancer Study V

Perioperative (Periop) therapy (begin within 36 h after mastectomy):

Cyclophosphamide	400 mg/m^2 i. v.	
Methotrexate	40 mg/m^2 i. v.	days 1 and 8
5-Fluorouracil	600 mg/m^2 i. v.	
Leucovorin[a]	15 mg i. v. 24 h after day 1 and 15 mg p. o. 24 h after day 8	

Conventionally timed adjuvant therapy (begins 25–32 days after mastectomy):

Cyclophosphamide	100 mg/m^2 orally	days 1–14	
Methotrexate	40 mg/m^2 i. v.	days 1 and 8	
5-Fluorouracil	600 mg/m^2 i. v.	days 1 and 8	Every 28 days
Prednisone	7.5 mg orally	daily	
Tamoxifen	20 mg orally	daily	

[a] Leucovorin added in January 1983

Trial Logistics

Assigned perioperative therapy must commence within 36 h of mastectomy. Thus, it was necessary to evolve a satisfactory system for rapid central registration and randomization. Randomization may occur immediately after mastectomy so that chemotherapy can be given on the first postoperative day, or prior to mastectomy and before a histological diagnosis has been obtained. If the patient's breast lesion is then found to be histologically benign, trial entry is canceled. Because of time zone differences, randomization is possible either in Bern, Switzerland, or in Sydney, Australia. Stratification is by clinic and menopausal status. Menopausal status is defined in Table 1.

Surgery

Total mastectomy with complete axillary clearance is the standard surgical procedure. This is carried out with or without removal of the pectoralis muscle(s). The protocol requires that all breast tissue be removed, a minimum of eight axillary lymph nodes be made available for histological examination, and that a specimen be prepared for estrogen receptor assay.

Eligibility Criteria

These include histologically confirmed breast cancer, a preoperative leukocyte count $\geqq 4000/mm^3$, a platelet count $\geqq 100000/mm^3$, serum creatinine $\leqq 1.5$ mg% or < 130 µmol/liter, bilirubin $\leqq 1.5$ mg% or $\leqq 20$ µmol/liter, serum glutamic oxaloacetic transaminase (SGOT $\leqq 60$ IU/liter, and a preoperative UICC performance status of 0-2. Patients who had prior therapy for breast cancer, who have other malignant disease, on whom a biopsy was performed more than 21 days prior to mastectomy, and who are surgical risks are ineligible for study entry.

Perioperative Chemotherapy (Immediately After Surgery)

The cytotoxic combination regimens which include cyclophosphamide (E), methotrexate (M), and 5-fluorouracil (F) are the ones most widely used and most often evaluated as adjuvant to surgery in breast cancer. This combination is therefore a logical choice for

Table 1. Menopausal status

Premenopausal and perimenopausal
>52 years and LNMP (last normal menstrual period) within 1 year, or
$\leqq 52$ years and LNMP within 3 years, or menstruating, or
$\leqq 55$ years and hysterectomy but no bilateral oophorectomy, or
Biochemical confirmation of continuing ovarian function (for doubtful patients)
Postmenopausal
>52 years with 1 year amenorrhea, or
$\leqq 52$ years with 3 years amenorrhea or more, or
Patients who have had hysterectomy without bilateral oophorectomy who are over 55 years, or
Biochemical evidence of cessation of ovarian function (for doubtful patients)

perioperative use in this study. The regimen includes: C, 400 mg/m^2 i.v.; M, 40 mg/m^2 i.v.; and F, 600 mg/m^2 i.v. on days 1 and 8. The intravenous route is chosen to ensure delivery and ease of administration in patients who have just undergone surgery. The perioperative chemotherapy (PeCT) is to be delivered within 36 h after mastectomy.

In November 1982, changes were made in this perioperative treatment because of unpredictable and severe toxic effects of the i.v. CMF regimen administered perioperatively (Ludwig Breast Cancer Study Group 1983). These changes were:

1. Leucovorin 15 mg i.v. was given 24 h after the first i.v. CMF dose and orally 24 h after the day 8 CMF administration.
2. Intravenous hydration for 36 h after mastectomy.
3. More stringent dose modification criteria were applied before giving i.v. CMF on day 8: (a) no drugs were given if any stomatitis was observed and (b) no methotrexate was given if day 8 serum creatinine was $\geqq$ 1.2 mg% ($\geqq$ 106 μmol/liter).
4. White blood cell count and platelet and serum creatinine determination were required on day 15.
5. Patients older than 65 years were excluded from entry into the trial.

It was suggested that the toxic effects observed in patients who had received i.v. CMF perioperatively were unpredictable due to interactions between nitrous oxide anesthesia and methotrexate. In fact, several published reports have drawn attention to the effects of nitrous oxide anesthesia on bone marrow function (Nunn et al. 1982; Deacon et al. 1980). It was suggested that nitrous oxide anesthesia might potentiate the toxicity of methotrexate by interfering with folate metabolism through inhibition of methionine synthetase (Kano et al. 1981). Moreover, nitrous oxide has been reported to reduce the motility of human neutrophils in vitro (Nunn and O'Morain 1982; Nunn et al. 1982), resulting in qualitative as well as quantitative granulocyte defects.[1]

At the beginning of 1984 we analyzed data on 690 evaluable patients who received perioperative chemotherapy and 373 evaluable patients who did not receive perioperative chemotherapy. Of the 690 patients, 443 received i.v. CMF without leucovorin, while 247 patients received i.v. CMF with the alterations described above (including leucovorin). As described previously, four patients died postoperatively following treatment with i.v. CMF (Ludwig Breast Cancer Study Group 1983). Two additional patients have died in the postoperative period (both on day 16 postmastectomy) due to pulmonary embolism; one patient received i.v. CMF therapy with leucovorin, and the other received no immediate chemotherapy after mastectomy. The incidence of toxic effects reported in the postoperative phase is described in Table 2.

Toxic effects considered to be dangerous or potentially dangerous were denoted in our previous report as toxicity X. These were wound-healing difficulties (wound-healing delay beyond 4 weeks, dehiscence, necrosis, extensive hematoma or seroma, or wound infection requiring drainage or antibiotics); severe myelosuppression (white blood cell count 10^9/liter and/or platelet count 5×10^{10}/liter); systemic infection; and stomatitis. The incidence of toxicity X was 23% and 24%, without and with the protocol alterations (Table 3). The reduction of severe components of toxicity X and stomatitis were counterbalanced by an increased incidence of reported seroma. This might be an indication of the increased thoroughness in monitoring patients. The significant reduction in reported stomatitis (*P*,

1 Leucovorin (5-formyl tetrahydrofolate) was administered intravenously to avoid conversion of formyl tetrahydrofolate to methyl tetrahydrofolate, which requires methionine synthetase action for utilization (Dudman et al. 1982)

Table 2. Postoperative complications and chemotherapy-related toxic effect: the impact of the addition of leucovorin rescue and other protocol alterations

Toxic effects	Percentage of group					
	Perioperative chemotherapy				No perioperative chemotherapy	
	leucovorin ($n=443$)		With leucovorin ($n=247$)		($n=373$)	
Deaths	0.9%		0.4%		0.3%	
Toxic effects	Mild/ moderate	Severe[a]	Mild/ moderate	Severe[a]	Mild/ moderate	Severe[a]
Leucopenia	50	1.6	64	0.4	–	–
In patients with midcourse counts	63	2.2	71	0.5	–	–
Thrombocytopenia	5	1.6	2	0.4	–	–
Anemia	7	1.6	7	0.4	–	–
Eye disorders (conjunctivitis)	2	0	1.2	0	–	–
Nausea and Vomiting	65	0.2	69	3.2	–	–
Diarrhea	4	0	4	0	–	–
Stomatitis	12	1.6	8	0.4	–	–
Renal impairment	0.7	0.2	0.4	0	–	–
Cystitis	1.4	0	0.4	0	–	–
Liver impairment	0.2	0.2	0.4	0	–	–
Depression	0.7	0	2	0	–	–
Alopecia	10	[b]	10	[b]	–	–
Postoperative Complications Infection systemic	2	1.4	3.6	0.8	0	0.3
Thrombophlebitis, thrombosis	1.6	0.5	0	1.2	0	0.3
Dehiscence of wound	3	0.9	3	0	0.8	0
Necrosis	1.1	0.2	1.2	0.8	1.1	0.5
Local infection	6	1.1	5	0	2.7	0.5
Seroma	6	0	15	0	6	0.3
Hematoma	1.8	0.2	1.6	0	1	0.3
Local hemorrhage	0	0.2	0.4	0	0	0.3
At least one postoperative complication	16.5	2.9	23.5	2.8	9.9	2.1
At least one of the above	79	7.0	83	6.5	9.9	2.1

[a] Severe: leukopenia $< 10^9$/liter; thrombocytopenia $< 5 \times 10^{10}$/liter; intractable nausea and vomiting; stomatitis ulcers, cannot eat; anemia with symptoms requiring transfusions; infection requiring antibiotics, surgery; renal impairment, $> 3\times$ normal creatinine; liver impairment, $>$ $5\times$ normal function tests; wound-healing problems, necrosis, local infection, hematoma requiring surgery for healing

[b] Not considered a severe effect

Table 3. Components of toxicity X

	i.v. CMF (%)	i.v. CMF+ leucovorin (%)
Overall toxicity X	23%	24%
Stomatitis	13%	8%
Leukopenia (10^9/liter)	2%	0.4%
Systemic infection	3%	4%
Wound healing	10%[a]	15%[b]

[a] Seroma alone accounts for 3% of this 10% incidence
[b] Seroma alone accounts for 7% of this 15% incidence

Table 4. Ludwig Breast Study V: Patient entry by institution November 81 - December 84

Institution	No. of patients
Auckland	66
Brescia	63
Cape Town	113
Essen/Düsseldorf	146
Göteborg	491
Ljubljana	147
Madrid	52
Melbourne	210
Perth	93
Sydney	80
Swiss Group (SAKK)	407
Total	1968

0.03) despite this improved monitoring indicated that the protocol alterations had reduced the mucosal toxicity possibly related to the postulated interaction between nitrous oxide anesthesia and methotrexate.

In our previous report we indicated that older patients ($\geqq 50$ years) and patients who started chemotherapy within 6 h from the end of mastectomy had higher rates of toxicity X. Patients 50 years or older who received CMF plus leucovorin continued to have more reported toxicity X than younger patients (29% versus 18%; *P*, 0.07). As only eight patients who received CMF plus leucovorin started chemotherapy within 6 h from the end of mastectomy, it was not possible to assess the impact of leucovorin upon the incidence of methotrexate-related toxicity within this group of patients in whom a methotrexate-nitrous oxide interaction might be expected (only one of the eight experienced wound-healing problems).

The changes in reported toxic effects could not be explained by the fact that more younger patients were entered into the trial after the protocol alterations. Moreover, there was no reduction in the average amount of CMF given, with or without leucovorin.

As an objective measure of desirable toxicity, we considered leucopenia for patients with midcourse white blood counts monitored. Seventy-two percent of the patients who received i.v. CMF without leucovorin had midcourse counts as compared with 86% who received the drug regimen with leucovorin. There was no significant change in the incidence of overall leucopenia (see Table 2); however, a slight reduction in the incidence of severe leucopenia was observed.

In this trial, in which one-third of the patients received the immediate postmastectomy chemotherapy as the only adjuvant treatment given, a desirable toxicity (Carpenter et al. 1982) could be achieved after alteration of the protocol without exposing the patient to the unpredictable toxic effects previously observed. A complete evaluation of the toxic effects will be made at the conclusion of accrual.

Conventionally Timed Adjuvant Therapy

The justification for using CMF is largely historical. Low-dose prednisone is added because of the data derived from the Toronto trial (Meakin et al. 1983) and because of the Group's own data showing that higher eytotoxic doses are tolerated with this agent. Tamoxifen is included in the postmenopausal regimen because of the higher response rate in conjunction with combination chemotherapy in advanced disease and because of positive results in several adjuvant trials (Deacon et al. 1980; Fisher et al. 1981). The 6-month duration of this "portion" of adjuvant treatment is based upon reports from Milan and Switzerland (Bonadonna et al. 1981; Jungi et al. 1981).

Pathology Central Review

A pathology central review laboratory is established for evaluation of the diagnosis, classification, and grading of the primary tumor and evaluation of the nontumor breast tissue and local or regional spread found in the biopsy and/or mastectomy specimen, including the axillary lymph nodes. Determination of treatment is based upon the evaluation of lymph node involvement by the responsible pathologist of the participating institution.

Hormone Receptor Determination

Determination of estrogen receptor and progesterone receptor in the tumor tissue is standardized and quality controlled on a groupwide basis.

Patient Accrual

As of December 1984, 1968 patients had been randomized into the trial (Table 4). Each treatment arm needs 550 patients with axillary node involvement to ensure the statistical validity of the results. An evaluation of the treatment results will be conducted when all patients are off treatment.

Comment

This report is of an informative character only. Conclusions, even with respect to the data on toxic effects, may be drawn only after the final evaluation. This will be made after completion of accrual and treatment of the last patient entered into the trial.

Ludwig Breast Cancer Study Group

Institution	
Ludwig Institute for Cancer Research Inselspital, Bern, Switzerland	A. Goldhirsch *(Study Coordinator)*, B. Davis, R. Bettelheim, W. Hartmann, *(Study Pathologists)*, D. Zava, C. Ramminger, C. Wiedmer
Harvard School of Public Health and Dana-Farber Cancer Center, Boston, USA	R. Gelber *(Study Statistician)*, K. Price, M. Zelen
Frontier Science & Technical Research Foundation, Buffalo, USA	M. Isley, M. Parsons, L. Szymoniak
Auckland Breast Cancer Study Group, Auckland, New Zealand	R. G. Kay, J. Probert, B. Mason, H. Wood, E. G. Gifford, J. F. Carter, J. C. Gillmann, J. Anderson, L. Yee, I. M. Holdaway, G. D. Hitchock, M. Jagusch
Spedali Civili & Fondazione Beretta, Brescia, Italy	G. Marini, E. Simoncini, P. Marpicati, U. Sartori, A. Barni, L. Morassi, P. Grigolato, D. Di Lorenzo, A. Albertini, G. Marinone, M. Zorzi
Groote Schuur Hospital, Cape Town, Republic of South Africa	A. Hacking, D. M. Dent, J. Terblanche, A. Tiltmann, A. Gudgeon, E. Dowdle, R. Sealy, P. Palmer
University of Essen, West German Tumor Center, Essen, Federal Republic of Germany	C. G. Schmidt, F. Schuning, K. Hoffken, L. D. Leder, H. Ludwig, R. Callies
University of Düsseldorf, Düsseldorf, Federal Republic of Germany	P. Faber, H. Bender, H. Bojar, H. G. Schnurch
West Swedish Breast Cancer Study Group, Göteborg, Sweden	C.-M. Rudenstam, E. Cahlin, H. Salander, I. Branehog, G. Jaderstrom, R. Hultborn, U. Wanneholt, S. Nilsson, J. Fornander, J. Save-Soderbergh, Ch. Johnsen, O. Ruusvik, G. Ostberg, L. Mattsson, C. G. Backstrom, S. Bergegardh, U. Ljungqvist, I. Dahl, Y. Hessman, S. Holmberg, S. Dahlin, G. Wallin
The Institute of Oncology, Ljubljana, Yugoslavia	J. Lindtner, J. Novak, M. Sencar, J. Cervek, O. Cerar, B. Stabuc, R. Golouh, J. Lamovec, J. Jancar, S. Sebek
Madrid Breast Cancer Group, Madrid, Spain	H. Cortes-Funes, F. Martinez-Tello, F. Cruz Caro, M. L. Marcos, M. A. Figueras, F. Calero, A. Suarez, F. Pastrana, R. Huertas
Anti-Cancer Council of Victoria, Melbourne, Australia	J. Collins, R. Snyder, R. Bennett, J. Burns, J. F. Forbes, J. Funder, E. Guli, L. Harrison, S. Hart, P. Kitchen, R. Lovell, R. Reed, I. Russell, A. Shaw, L. Sisely, R. D. Snyder, P. Jeal, J. H. Colebatch
Sir Charles Gairdner Hospital Nedlands, Western Australia, Australia	M. Byrne, P. M. Reynolds, H. J. Sheiner, S. Levitt, D. Kermode, K. B. Shilkin, R. Hahnel
SAKK Swiss Group for Clinical Cancer Research Bern, Inselspital, Switzerland	K. Brunner, M. Berger, H. Cottier, G. Locher, K. Burki, E. Dreher, M. Walther, M. Castiglione, R. Joss, A. Pedrazzini, U. Herrmann, P. Herrmann
St. Gallen, Kantonsspital, Switzerland	W. F. Jungi, H. J. Senn, A. Mutzner, U. Schmidt, Th. Hardmeier, E. Hochuli, O. Schildknect

Ludwig Breast Cancer Study Group *(continued)*

Institution	
Bellinzona, Ospedal San Giovanni, Switzerland	F. Cavalli, M. Varini, P. Luscieti, E. S. Passega, G. Losa
Basel, Kantonsspital, Switzerland	J. P. Obrecht, F. Harder, A. C. Almendral, U. Eppenberger, J. Torhorst
Geneva, Hopital Cantonal Universitaire, Switzerland	P. Alberto, F. Krauer, R. Egeli, R. Megevand, M. Forni, P. Schafer, E. Jacot des Combes, A. M. Schindler, F. Misset
Lausanne, Centre Hospitalier Universitaire Vaudois, Switzerland	S. Leyvraz
Neuchatel, Hopital des Cadolles, Switzerland	P. Siegenthaler, V. Barrelet, R. P. Baumann
Lucerne, Kantonsspital, Switzerland	H. J. Schmid
Ludwig Institute for Cancer Research and Royal Prince Alfred Hospital, Sydney, Australia	M. H. N. Tattersall, R. Fox, A. Coates, D. Hedley, D. Raghavan, F. Niesche, R. West, S. Renwick, D. Green, J. Donovan, P. Duval, A. Ng, T. Foo, D. Glenn, T. J. Nash, R. A. North, J. Beith, G. O'Connor
Wellington Hospital, New Zealand	J. S. Simpson

References

Bonadonna G, Valagussa P (1981) Dose-response effect of adjuvant chemotherapy in breast cancer. N Engl J Med 304: 15-20

Bonadonna G, Valagussa P, Rossi A, Zucali R, Tancini G, Bajetta E, Brambilla C, DeLena M, Di-Fronzo G, Banfi A, Rilke F, Veronesi U (1978) Are surgical adjuvant trials altering the course of breast cancer? Semin Oncol 5: 450-464

Bonadonna G, Rossi A, Tancini G, Brambilla C, Marchini S, Valagussa P, Veronesi U (1981) Adjuvant treatment for breast cancer: the Milan Institute experience (1981) Proc 3rd International conference on the adjuvant therapy of cancer, Tucson, Arizona, March 18-21

Carpenter TT, Maddox WA, Laws HL, Wirtschafter DD, Soong SJ (1982) Favorable factors in the adjuvant therapy of breast cancer. Cancer 50: 18-23

Deacon R, Lumb M, Perry J (1980) Inactivation of methionine synthetase by nitrous oxide. Eur J Biochem 104: 419-422

Dewys WD (1972) Studies correlating the growth rate of a tumor and its metastases and providing evidence for tumor-related systemic growth-retarding factors. Cancer Res 32: 374-379

Dudman NPB, Slowiaczek P, Tattersall MHN (1982) Methotrexate rescue by 5-methyl THF in lymphoblastoid cell lines. Cancer Res 42: 502-507

Fisher B, Slack NH, Katrych D, Wolmark N (1975) Ten years of follow-up results of patients with carcinoma of the breast in a cooperative clinical trial evaluating surgical adjuvant chemotherapy. Surg Gynecol Obstet 140: 528-534

Fisher B, Redmond C, Brown A (1981) Treatment of primary breast cancer with chemotherapy and tamoxifen. N Engl J Med 305: 1-6

Fisher B, Gunduz N, Saffer EA (1983) Influence of the interval between primary tumor removal and chemotherapy on kinetics and growth of metastases. Cancer Res 43: 1488-1492

Goldie JH, Coldman AJ (1979) A mathematical model for relating the drug sensitivity of tumors to their spontaneous mutation rate. Cancer Treat Rep 63: 1727-1733

Hubay CA, Pearson OH, Marshall JS, Stellato TA, Rhodes RS, DeBanne SM, Rosenblatt J, Mansour EG, Hermann RE, Jones JC, Flynn WJ, Eckert C, McGuire WL (1981) Antiestrogen, cytotox-

ic chemotherapy and bacillus Calmette-Guerin vaccination in stage II breast cancer: a preliminary report. Surgery 87: 494-501
Joint BCTC/WHO/UICC Overview (1984) Overview of mortality results in randomized trials in early breast cancer. Lancet ii: 1205
Jungi WF, Brunner KW, Cavalli F, Martz G, Rosset G, Barrelet L (1981) Short- or long-term adjuvant chemotherapy for breast cancer. Proc Am Assoc Cancer Res ASCO 22: 435 (Abstract C-399)
Kano Y, Sakamoto S, Sakuraya K, Kubota T, Hida K, Suda K, Takaku F (1981) Effect of nitrous oxide on human bone marrow cells and its synergistic effect with methionine and methotrexate on functional folate deficiency. Cancer Res 41: 4698-4701
Ludwig Breast Cancer Study Group (1983) Toxic effects of early adjuvant chemotherapy for breast cancer. Lancet ii: 542-544
Meakin JW, Allt WEC, Beale FA, Bush RS, Clark RN and other PMH and ICRF investigators (1983) Ovarian irradiation and prednisone following surgery and radiotherapy for carcinoma of the breast. Breast Cancer Res Treatment 3: 45-48
Nissen-Meyer R, Kjellgren K, Malmio K. Mansson B, Norin T (1978) Surgical adjuvant chemotherapy: results with one short course with cyclophosphamide after mastectomy for breast cancer. Cancer 41: 2088-2098
Nunn JF, O'Morain C (1982) Nitrous oxide decreases motility of human neutrophils in vitro. Anesthesiology 56: 45-48
Nunn JF, Sharer NM, Gorchein A, Jones JA, Wickranasinghe SN (1982) Megaloblastic hemopoiesis after multiple short-term exposure to nitrous oxide. Lancet i: 1379-1381
Schabel FM (1977) Surgical adjuvant chemotherapy of metastatic murine tumors. Cancer 40: 558-568

Neoadjuvant Chemotherapy in the Conservative Management of Breast Cancers: Study of 143 Patients

C. I. Jacquillat, M. Weil, G. Auclerc, M. Sellami, M. F. Auclerc, D. Khayat, and F. Baillet

Service d'Oncologie Médicale Hôpital de la Salpétrière, 47 Boulevard de l'Hôpital, 75013 Paris Cedex 13, France

Introduction

Our thinking concerning breast cancer has evolved considerably over the past 10 years. The concept of a local disease with secondary metastases has given way to that of a two-component disease, local and systemic. The larger the tumor size, the faster the growth rate, the lesser the degree of differentiation of the tumor, and the greater the lymph node involvement; these are the factors which characterize the disease.

Although patients with localized breast cancer have a 5-year survival that varies between 65% and 85%, 80% will die from their cancer within 20 years of the primary diagnosis (Ferguson et al. 1982).

Theoretical (Goldie and Coldman 1979), experimental (Karrer et al. 1967; Schabel et al. 1979), and clinical data (Nissen-Meyer et al. 1978; Fisher 1982) have indicated that chemotherapy should be used at the earliest possible time. Neoadjuvant chemotherapy not only improves the effect of local treatment with surgery or radiotherapy and ensures the early treatment of micrometastases but also enables the activity of a given drug regimen to be assessed in individual patients by measuring the degree of tumor regression.

The local treatment chosen in this study was radiotherapy. It had already been demonstrated that the 10-year survival achieved with exclusive irradiation is similar to that obtained by standard surgical procedures. It was also shown, for patients with T2 and T3 lesions with no prior tumorectomy, that the combination of external and endocurietherapy with irridium-192 gives a much higher rate of breast conservation (Otmezguine et al. 1980).

Material and Methods

Between 1 January 1980 and 1 January 1985, 143 patients were entered on study S180 combining primary chemotherapy, locoregional radiotherapy, and maintenance chemotherapy with or without hormonotherapy. All patients had a complete history and physical examination, complete blood counts, serum chemistry and carcinoembryonic antigen determination, urinalysis, electrocardiogram and echocardiogram, chest roentgenograms, bone scan, liver echography, and bilateral mammograms. Diagnosis relied on aspiration cytology and histology obtained by drill biopsy. As shown in Table 1, patients were stratified into four groups according to clinical stage; their age distribution is shown in Table 2. The criteria of locally advanced breast cancer were fulfilled in 83 patients: all patients in groups III and IV and 13 patients in group II with tumor diameters over 5 cm (Canellos 1984).

Recent Results in Cancer Research. Vol 103

Table 1. Patient classification by group

Group		Stage	Number of patients[a]	Total
I		T1 N0	6	
		T2 N0	15	24
		N1a	3	
II		T1 N1b	1	
		T2 N0	20	
		N1a	5	
		N1b	10	49
		T3 N0	4	
		N1a	5	
		N1b	4	
III		T3 N0	7	
		N1a	2	16
		N1b	3	
		N2	4	
IV		T4 N0	3	
		N1b	6	
		N2	3	
	PeV1[b]	T3 N0	6	
		T3 N1a	3	
		T3 N1b	2	
		T4 N1b	1	
	PeV2[b]	T1 N1b	1	
		T2 cN2	1	
		T3 N0	1	54
		T3 N1a	3	
		T3 N1b	10	
		T4 N0	3	
		T4 N1b	5	
		T4 N2	1	
	PeV3[b]	T3 N2	1	
		T4 N0	2	
		T4 N1b	1	
		T4 N3	1	
Total				143

[a] In eight patient interstitial radiotherapy was not completed
[b] PeV1, clinical doubling time less than 6 weeks
PeV2, inflammatory signs limited to a part of the breast
PeV3, inflammatory signs involving the whole breast

Initial treatment consisted of the intravenous infusion of the combination of vinblastine (6 mg/m^2), thiotepa (6 mg/m^2), methotrexate (25 mg/m^2), and 5-fluorouracil (350 mg/m^2) given over 1 h (VTMF), to which Adriamycin (30 mg/m^2) was added for group III and IV patients (VTMFA).

Local treatment consisted of teleradiotherapy to the breast and regional lymph nodes, administered according to the classical schedule in group I and II patients (45 grays with-

Table 2. Age distribution of patients by groups

Age (years)	Group				Total
	I	II	III	IV	
20–29	–	–	1	3	4
30–39	3	1	2	12	18
40–49	4	15	4	17	40
50–59	7	19	7	14	47
60–75	10	14	2	8	34
Total	24	49	16	54	143

in 5 weeks) and in two bimonthly courses of two consecutive days in group III and IV patients. An infusion of chemotherapy without methotrexate and Adriamycin was interspaced between the split-course of irradiation; 2 weeks later, after another chemotherapy dose, a boost to the initial tumor site by means of endocurietherapy with irridium-192 was administered (30 grays). Thereafter maintenance chemotherapy with the same combination was given for 5 monthly cycles for group I, for 6 bimonthly cycles followed by 12 monthly cycles for group II, and for 6 bimonthly cycles followed by 6 cycles every 3 weeks and then by 12 monthly cycles for groups III and IV. Adriamycin was stopped after a cumulative dose of 300 mg/m^2. In addition, tamoxifen (TMX) was given to all menopausal patients; premenopausal patients received this drug by random allocation.

Results

As shown in Table 3, initial chemotherapy induced a tumor regression of over 50% in 124 patients (87%) with complete remissions occurring in 26 cases (18%). Partial remissions were further obtained in 38 patients after external radiotherapy. In all cases, tumor regression became complete 3 months after the end of interstitial irradiation. In groups I and II a survival rate of 100% was achieved (median follow-up of 24 months) with a disease-free survival at 4 years of 81% (Fig. 1). In these groups, only two local recurrences requiring mastectomy and three metastatic relapses occurred.

Table 3. Number of patients with indicated tumor regression after primary therapy

Regression after	Percentage Regression <25	26–50	51–75	76–99	100
1. Chemotherapy					
Group I	8	2	7	8	5
Group II	4	3	14	20	8
Group III	0	2	2	8	4
Group IV	2	4	14	25	9
Total	14	11	37	61	26
				87% (51–100)	
2. External irradiation	–	2	8	30	103
3. Interstitial irradiation					143

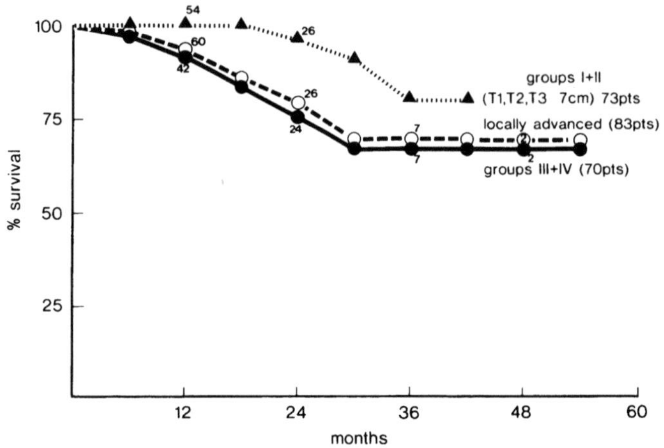

Fig. 1. Percentage 4-year survival of groups I and II and groups III and IV

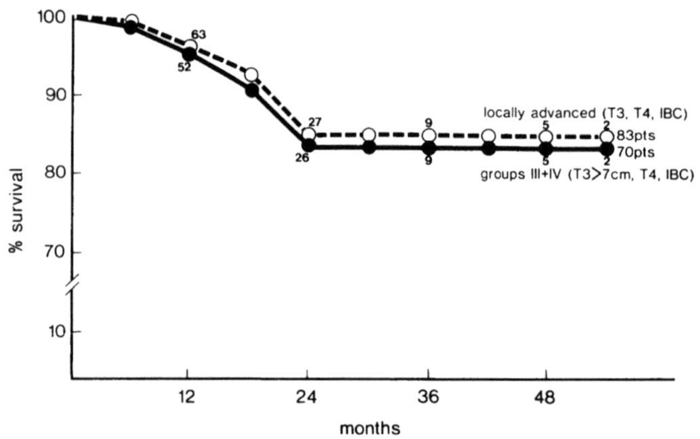

Fig. 2. Percentage 3-year survival of groups I and II and groups III and IV

Of the 70 patients belonging to groups III and IV, 7 died from metastases within the first 2 years (metastases were preceded by local relapses requiring mastectomy in two of these patients), 2 are alive and in complete remission after local relapses that required mastectomy, and 2 have active metastases. In these groups a 3-year survival of 85% and a disease-free survival of 72% were observed (Fig. 2).

A relationship between the degree of initial tumor regression and outcome was noted. As shown in Table 4, the frequency of recurrence was 20% in the 56 patients whose initial tumor regression was less than 75%, compared with 8% in the 87 patients with tumor regression greater than 75%. The pattern of first relapses and their relationship to initial regression are shown in Table 5.

Comparing the 83 patients who received TMX to the 55 patients who did not, initial tumor regression over 75% was more frequent in the TMX-treated group although the difference was not statistically significant. Similarly, the relapse rate was not significantly reduced in TMX-treated patients. Random allocation in premenopausal patients was not always respected, however.

Table 4. Frequency of relapse in relation to tumor regression after chemotherapy

Regression (%)	Relapse	
≦ 25	2/ 8	
26– 50	3/11	11/56 (20%)
51– 75	7/37	
		$P<0.01$
76– 99	1/61	7/87 (8%)
100	5/26	

Table 5. Pattern of relapses in relation to initial tumor regression

Patient group	Clinical stage	Percentage regression[a]	Relapse			Months of follow-up (*A*, alive; *D*, dead)
			Local	Distant	Months from diagnosis	
I	T2 N0	40	–	Bone	17	34 (A)
	T2 N1a	70	–	Eye	42	43 (A)
II	T2 N1b	66	+	–	24	27 (A)
	T2 N0	?	–	Bone	15	16 (A)
	T2 N0	70	+	–	20	21 (A)
III	T3 N1b	10	+	–	17	22 (D)
	T3 N0	0	–	Bone marrow, liver	4	5 (D)
	T3 N3	100	+	–	16	21 (D)
IV	T3 N1b PeV3	100	–	Liver	6	9 (D)
	T4 N1b	100	–	Bone, liver	30	44 (A)
	T4 N0	78	+	–	27	38 (A)
	T3 N2 PeV2	42	+	–	22	30 (A)
	T3 N1b PeV2	51	–	Bone	6	15 (D)
	T3 N1b PeV1	58	–	Bone	14	16 (D)
	T3 N1b PeV1	100	–	Liver	24	29 (A)
	T2 N2 PeV2	100	–	Bone	13	21 (A)
	T3 N1b PeV2	58	–	Bone marrow	22	22 (D)
	T4b N0 PeV3	75	–	Bone	8	15 (A)

[a] Regression after initial chemotherapy

Toxicity

Clinical toxicity was dominated by nausea, asthenia, and alopecia. In most patients, hospitalization was restricted to the 3 days required by endocurietherapy. In groups I and II, hematological toxicity (less than 1000 neutrophils/mm^3, and/or less than 100000 platelets/mm^3) did not require any treatment modification. In groups III and IV one or two cycles of chemotherapy had to be delayed, thus lengthening the period of induction therapy (Table 6). One patient (group IV) with a family history of acute leukemia died of acute myelocytic leukemia at 24 months. At the time of writing, the cosmetic results have been excellent in the majority of patients.

Table 6. Hematological toxicity

	Rating	% Dose given	Treatment spread (weeks)
Group I	1	95	-
Group II	1	97	-
Group III	2	95	5,6 instead of 4
Group IV	2-3	92	7 instead of 6

Discussion

Our study confirms the effectiveness of a combined-modality approach using neoadjuvant chemotherapy and radiotherapy in the treatment of patients with breast cancer. Tumor regression of over 50% was observed in 87% of patients. Despite the large initial tumor burden observed in 83 patients with locally advanced breast cancer, the regression induced by chemotherapy allowed conservative treatment of the breast in most patients since only six local relapses required secondary mastectomies.

In groups III and IV the 4-year disease-free overall survivals were 70% and 83%, respectively. These results are in keeping with those reported by other authors (Chauvergne et al. 1979; Papaioannou 1981; Zylberberg et al. 1982; Kantarjian et al. 1984) and represent a significant improvement over historical controls (Rubens et al. 1980). We also observed a significant correlation between the degree of initial tumor regression and the distant outcome. The primary use of cytoreductive chemotherapy until maximal tumor regression is achieved before instituting local therapy seems, therefore, appropriate. The optimal timing of radiotherapy would depend on the tumor burden and chemosensitivity.

An unsettled question concerns the optimal use of combination chemotherapy and hormonotherapy. In this study, hormonal receptor studies were not available in most patients. The precise level of receptors below which hormonotherapy is inactive, as well as the best combination schedule, remains unknown.

Another unsolved problem is the optimum duration of maintenance chemotherapy. Randomized studies, such as the one carried out by Tancini (Tancini et al. 1983), are obviously necessary to answer this question.

In conclusion, the use of a combined treatment modality consisting of neoadjuvant chemotherapy and maintenance therapy in addition to teleradiotherapy and endocurietherapy allowed breast conservation in 136/142 patients.

For patients with initial tumors over 7 cm (13 pts) and for inflammatory breast cancers (54 pts), the 4-year disease-free survival and overall survival rates are 70% and 83%, respectively. Increased understanding of the natural history of breast cancers and more refined knowledge about drugs pharmacology and tumor cells resistance will further improve the prognosis of this disease.

Acknowledgements. The study was supported by INSERM and CRAC (Centre de recherches appliquées à la chimiothérapie). The authors are thankful to Dr. Amina Jindani for her help in the translation and to Brigitte Cedreau for her excellent technical assistance.

References

Canellos GP (1984) The treatment of locally advanced breast cancer. J Clin Oncol 2: 149-151

Chauvergne J, Durand M, Hoerni B, Cohen P, Lagard C (1979) La chimiothérapie d'induction dans les cancers du sein à haut risque. Résultats d'une étude thérapeutique prospective. Bull Cancer 66: 9-16

Fergusson DJ, Meier P, Karrison J, Dawson PJ, Straus FH, Lowenstein FG (1982) Staging of breast cancer and survival rates. JAMA 248: 1337-1341

Fisher F, Redmond C, Elias G, Evans J, et al (1982) Adjuvant chemotherapy of breast cancer: an overview of NSABP findings. Adv Surg Oncol 5: 65-90

Goldie JH, Coldman AJ (1979) A mathematical model for relating the drug sensitivity of tumors to their spontaneous mutation rate. Cancer Treat Rep 63: 1727-1733

Kantarjian HP, Hortobagyi GN, Smith TL, Blumenschein GR, Montague E, Buzdar AU, Martin RG (1984) The management of locally advanced breast cancer a combined modality approach. Eur J Cancer Clin Oncol 20: 1353-1361

Karrer K, Humphreys SR, Goldin A (1967) An experimental model for studying factors which influence metastases of malignant tumors. Int J Cancer 2: 213-223

Nissen-Meyer R, Kjellgren K, Malmio K, Mansson B, Norin T (1978) Surgical adjuvant chemotherapy: results of one short course with cyclophosphamide after mastectomy for breast cancer. Cancer 41: 2088-2098

Otmezguine Y, Martin A, Le Bourgeois JP, Maylin C, Raynal M, Sallé M, Pierquin B (1980) Etude des récidives parmi 202 cancéreuses du sein traitées conservativement par radiothérapie. J Eur Radiother 1: 115-130

Papaioannou AN (1981) Preoperative chemotherapy for operable breast cancer. Eur J Cancer 17: 263-269

Powell K, Buzdar A, Smith T, Blumenschein G (1982) Subsequent malignant neoplasms in stage II, III breast cancer patients treated with and without adjuvant combination chemotherapy (meeting abstract). Proc Am Soc Clin Oncol 1: 78 (C301)

Rubens RD, Seston S, Tong D (1980) Combined chemotherapy and radiotherapy for locally advanced breast cancer. Eur J Cancer 16: 351-356

Schabel FM, Griswold DP, Corbett TH, Laster Jr, Dykes DJ, Rose WC (1979) Recent studies with adjuvant chemotherapy or immunotherapy of metastatic solid tumors of mice. In: Jones SE, Salmon SE (eds) Adjuvant therapy of cancer. Grune and Stratton, New York, pp 3-17

Tancini G, Bonadonna G, Valagussa P, et al. (1983) Adjuvant CMF in breast cancer comparative 5-year results of 12 versus 6 cycles. J Clin Oncol 1: 1-10

Zylberberg B, Salat-Baroux J, Ravina JH, Dormont D, Amiel JP, Diebold P, Izrael V (1982) Initial chemoimmunotherapy in inflammatory carcinoma of the breast. Cancer 49: 1537-1543

Preliminary Results of Preoperative Chemotherapy with a Combination of Platinum-Bleomycin Administered in 5-Day Cycles in Carcinoma of the Bronchus

J. Clavier, L. Israël, G. Nouvet, Y. Raut, J.-J. Gres, J.-F. Morère, C. Zabbe, G. Lerebours-Pigeonnière, and J.-L. Breau

Hôpital Augustin Morvan, Service de Pneumologie, CHR de Brest, 29279 Brest, France

Introduction

The results obtained with local treatments for inoperable squamous carcinomas of the lung (surgery with or without radiotherapy) depend solely on the stage of the tumor at the time of the operation and have been the same for several decades. We decided to conduct a preliminary, nonrandomized trial of preoperative chemotherapy in these cases because of: (1) the stable and reproducible nature of the postoperative survival curves which enable us to evaluate, if not measure, any possible therapeutic benefit, (2) the effectiveness of 5-day cycles of the combination of platinum-bleomycin in the histological group of squamous carcinomas (Israel et al. 1981 a, 1981 b; Elson et al. 1982), (3) the possible importance of the DNA repair process in the clinical resistance of these cancers and the role of the above combination in the inhibition of these processes (Okuyama and Mishina 1980; Israel et al. 1985).

Population Treated

One hundred and eleven male subjects with squamous bronchial carcinoma were studied. Their age ranged from 35 to 73 years (median 56 years).

In each case, the diagnosis was established by means of bronchial biopsy. Each patient was also investigated by means of mediastinal tomography and/or CT scan and by respiratory function tests. Mediastinoscopy was performed in 12 cases. The presurgical staging was as follows:

Stage I	60 cases
Stage II	12 cases
Stage III	39 cases

In 43 cases in this series (34 stage III and 9 stage II), the surgeon initially decided that the patient was inoperable either for functional reasons or, more importantly, in 40 cases, for anatomical reasons, such as bronchial extension or parietal or mediastinal involvement.

Modalities of treatment

1. Treatment consisted of two to four cycles of preoperative chemotherapy with the platinum-bleomycin combination, with the addition of mitomycin-C in nine cases and vindesine in seven cases.

Recent Results in Cancer Research. Vol 103

Platinum was administered for five consecutive days, every 3 weeks, at a dose of 20 mg/m^2 per day and at a rate of 1 mg/min, after suitable hydration of the patient. Calcium and magnesium were administered during and after treatment until the time of operation. Creatinine clearance was studied prior to each treatment and platinum was withheld for values below 70 ml/min. Methylprednisolone 120 mg was administered with each treatment in order to prevent nausea and vomiting (Breau et al. 1983).

Bleomycin was administered in the form of a continuous infusion at a dose of 5 mg/m^2 per day, 24 h a day, in 500 ml glucose saline for a period of 5 days. The CO diffusion was measured prior to each cycle and bleomycin was withheld if this value decreased by 25% in relation to the initial value (after correction of anemia and after optimal treatment of bronchial obstruction).

The treatment cycles were repeated every 21 days and the operation was performed 2 weeks after the end of the last course of chemotherapy. The anesthetic involved the use of a mixture of 50% nitrogen-oxygen and not pure oxygen.

Chest X-rays and a full blood count were also performed prior to each cycle and prior to the operation. Bronchoscopy was performed preoperatively in the cases initially considered to be inoperable by the surgeon and in the cases of apparent complete remission.

2. Postoperative therapy for cases evaluated to be N1 after the operation consisted of irradiation only in the form of 46 grays to the site of the tumor, the mediastinum, and the homolateral supraclavicular lymph nodes as well as an overdosage of 15 grays to the site of the tumor. In the cases evaluated to be N2, this radiotherapy was followed by chemotherapy consisting of a combination of platinum and vindesine for a maximum of six cycles, at a rhythm of one cycle every 4 weeks. The cases evaluated to be N− received no postoperative treatment.

Results of the Induction Treatment

1. Preoperative objective response consisted of at least a decrease by more than 50% in the product of the two perpendicular diameters of the measurable tumor on successive chest X-rays (excluding atelectasis). Complete responses consisted in the disappearance of the radiological image, with a completely normal endoscopic appearance and a negative bronchial biopsy. A decrease in the lesion of less than 50% was recorded as no change.
2. Preoperative evaluation of the results revealed: complete responses, 20; partial objective responses, 71; no change, 20; and tumor progression, 0. It should be noted that all of the complete responses were observed in cases considered to be stage I at the beginning of treatment.
3. The following surgical operations were performed: pneumonectomy, 53 cases; lobectomy, 47 cases; wedge resection, 5 cases; exploratory thoracotomy without resection, 6 cases.
4. In the 20 cases with preoperative complete response, histological examination of the operative specimen revealed complete disappearance of the tumor in 7 cases (i.e., 11.6% of the stage I cases) and almost complete disappearance in 6 cases.

Toxicity and Complications

1. Preoperative toxicity consisted of:
   a) Thirty percent incidence of gastrointestinal disturbances with nausea and vomiting due to platinum. These effects were treated by metoclopramide.
   b) Twelve cases of mild hematological toxicity in the patients treated with mitomycin C or vindesine.
   c) No cases of deterioration of the resiratory function.

   All of the eleven patients were suitable for surgery.
2. The postoperative complications observed within 30 days of the operation consisted of: pulmonary embolism, three cases; bronchial fistula, four cases; septic complications, three cases; massive hemoptysis, one case; and interstitial lung disease, one case.
3. The causes of deaths occurring within 2 months of the operation, during the course of radiotherapy, were as follows: pulmonary embolism, three cases; bronchial fistula, six cases; septic complications, six cases; massive hemoptysis, one case; and interstitial lung disease, six cases.
   It should be noted that the postoperative radiotherapy increased the number of cases of bronchial fistula, septic omplications, and interstitial lung disease. All of these additional complications occurred in patients who had received vindesine or mitomycin C in addition to the platinum-bleomycin combination.
4. The causes of deaths occurring beyond 2 months after the operation were as follows: locoregional recurrence, five cases; distant metastases, ten cases; causes unrelated to the cancer, nine cases.

Long-Term Survival

The follow-up of the 111 patients studied varied between 4 and 44 months with a mean follow-up of 10 months. The actuarial survival must therefore be interpreted very carefully.

As shown in Fig. 1, we can now accept that the median survival for patients with stage I cancer will exceed 45 months, with a plateau at the time of writing of 65% of the initial population. The projected median survival for patients with stage II cancer was 28 months, with a 3-year survival of 40%, while the projected median survival for stage III patients was 14 months with a projected survival of 12% at 45 months.

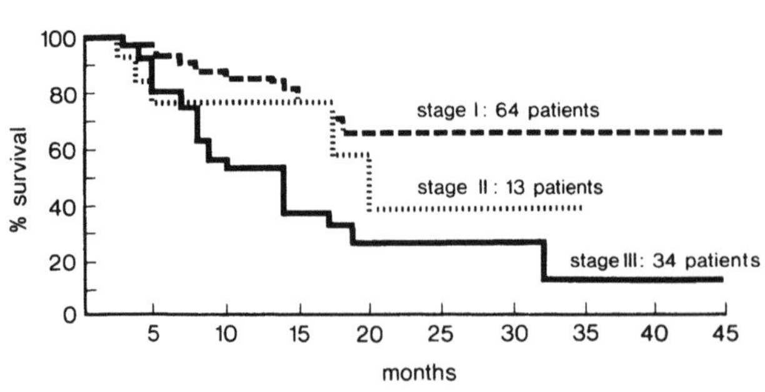

Fig. 1. Survival of patients with squamous cell lung carcinoma treated with preoperative chemotherapy

Discussion

1. The effectiveness and tolerance of the chemotherapy used could be improved. Toxicity evaluation indicated that the addition of mitomycin C or vindesine should be avoided as these drugs were probably responsible for some of the postoperative complications occurring before or during radiotherapy, and had a negative influence on the overall survival.
   A trial is currently in progress in cases judged inoperable, comparing the platinum-bleomycin combination with a platinum-bleomycin-VP16 combination administered in 5-day cycles. If this combination is found to be more effective, without any additional toxicity, it will be studied in the preoperative situation.
2. The results reported here demonstrate the feasibility of preoperative chemotherapy in squamous cell carcinomas of the bronchus, but they do not allow us to express an opinion on its effectiveness, for the following reasons: (a) a randomized trial is not available, but will be performed in the future; and (b) the results obtained do not appear to be superior to those reported in the absence of preoperative chemotherapy. However, more than one-third of the cases included in this preliminary study would normally have been considered to be inoperable and were subsequently rendered operable by the treatment.
   Future randomized trials should compare operable patients, stratified by stage, with or without preoperative chemotherapy with inoperable patients, all submitted to systematic chemotherapy and made operable by this treatment and subsequently randomized between surgery and continued medical treatment. The particular nature of the patients with squamous cell carcinoma of the bronchus, due to the proximity of the vital organs in the mediastinum and the coexistence of functional alterations of the respiratory system and the cardiovascular system, makes such comparisons very difficult.

References

Breau JL, Israël L, Pochmalicki G (1983) Efficacité de la méthylprednisolone dans la prévention des vomissements dus aux sels de platine dans un essai randomisé. Bull Cancer 70: 230

Elson DL, Holm ME, Reed RC (1982) Bleomycin infusion plus cisplatin effective induction therapy for squamous cell carcinoma. Proc ASCO 1: 147 (Abstract C-572)

Israël L, Aguilera J, Breau JL (1981 a) Traitement des cancers épidermoides par bléomycine et platine en administration continue prolongée. Série préliminaire de 80 cas avec 75% de réponses objectives. Nouv Presse Méd 10: 1817-1824

Israël L, Aguilera J, Breau JL (1981 b) Preliminary report of 70% response rate in squamous cell ca of the lung with a 6 consecutive days combination of cis-platinum bleomycin. Proc ASCO 1: 508 (Abstract C-685)

Israël L, Breau JL, Morère JF, Lepage E, Aguilera J (1985) Inhibition de la réparation de l'ADN, objectif majeur des chimiothérapies anticancéreuses. A propos de 680 cas de combinaison platine-bléomycine en continu. Ann Méd Int 1: 17-20

Okuyama S, Mishina H (1980) Consecutive therapy of cancer aimed at perpetuation of repairable damage: a hypothesis unifying radiotherapy and chemotherapy. J Clin Hematol Oncol 10: 83-93

Impact of Primary Site of Stage III and IV Squamous Cell Carcinomas of the Head and Neck on 7-Year Survival Figures Following Initial Non-Cisplatin-Containing Combination Chemotherapy

L. A. Price and B. T. Hill

Royal Marsden Hospital and Imperial Cancer Research Fund Laboratories,
Lincoln's Inn Fields, P.O. Box 123, London WC2A 3PX, Great Britain

Introduction

The traditional initial treatment of advanced squamous cell carcinomas of the head and neck with surgery and radiation remains unsatisfactory and continues to provide disappointing 5-year survival figures. Adjuvant chemotherapy has proved a useful addition to these local therapies in the treatment of many different "solid" tumors, with improved survival figures resulting from this combined modality approach in pediatric tumors, testicular teratomas, non-Hodgkin's lymphomas, sarcomas, and breast cancers (DeVita 1984). Similar approaches are now being applied to stage III, stage IV, and inoperable cancers of the head and neck region (for example: Hill et al. 1984; Hong et al. 1981; Kish et al. 1982, 1984; Perry et al. 1984; Price and Hill 1982; Price et al. 1983; Spaulding et al. 1982, 1983).

In 1973 we initiated a program with the objective of establishing the role of chemotherapy in advanced head and neck cancer. We first demonstrated, using a combination of seven standard drugs, that intensive chemotherapy could be given safely to these patients and that it was effective, resulting in a 70% response rate (Price et al. 1975). Next, we showed how a combination of vincristine, methotrexate, bleomycin, and 5-fluorouracil, with or without Adriamycin, could be integrated safely with radiotherapy and/or surgery, without requiring any modifications in their planned tretments (Price and Hill 1977). Furthermore, we established that the results with initial chemotherapy were significantly superior to those achieved using chemotherapy to treat recurrent or previously irradiated disease. Therefore in 1975 we set up a study to determine the impact of initial chemotherapy followed by local therapy on survival. Unfortunately we have not been able to carry out a randomized, controlled clinical study at the Royal Marsden Hospital. However, between January 1975 and December 1983, 178 patients with stage III and stage IV tumors of the head and neck have been entered into this study. In this large series we aimed to identify any particular subgroups of patients with tumors who derived definite survival benefit from this approach. We now report long-term 7-year survival data, providing evidence that response to this initial combination schedule A chemotherapy protocol is a good prognostic sign for overall survival, but only for tumors at certain sites.

Patients and Methods

One hundred and seventy-eight patients were entered into this study. One hundred and seventy-five patients were considered eligible with histologically proven squamous cell carcinomas of the head and neck. These patients had not received prior therapy of any kind and were judged free of metastases beyond the regional lymph nodes. No patients

Recent Results in Cancer Research. Vol 103

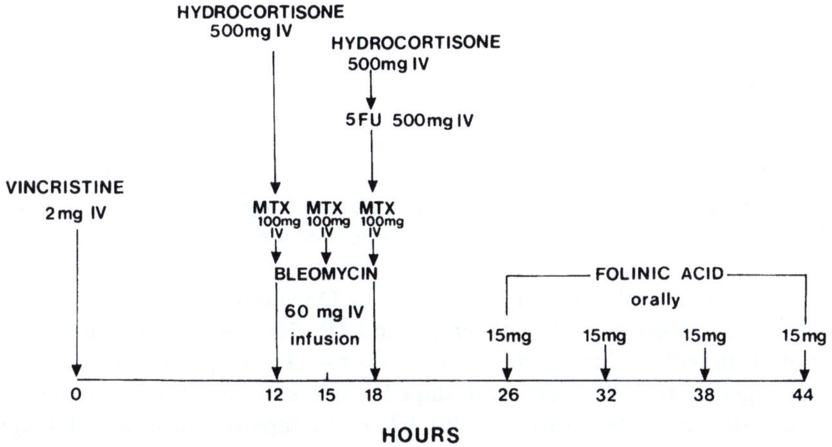

Fig. 1. Price-Hill schedule A chemotherapy protocol without cisplatin

Table 1. Medical precautions to be observed

1. All patients were carefully examined clinically and had full hematological and biochemical profiles
2. Another treatment cycle was *never* given unless the peripheral blood count had returned to its original level. If in doubt treatment was postponed for 1 week
3. Patients with impaired renal function were given a proportionately extended folinic acid rescue
4. All patients were hydrated so as to produce a urinary output of at least 2 liters over the 24-h treatment period. Patients with cardiovascular disease were given frusemide IV at the end of the bleomycin infusion
5. Bleomycin was omitted from the second course if it produced an acute reaction after the first treatment
6. Patients with a history of chronic respiratory disease were investigated for a diffusion defect. If one was found, bleomycin was omitted

were considered resectable for cure prior to chemotherapy. Seventy-one patients had stage IV tumors and 104 patients had stage III disease. Details of the combination chemotherapy schedule A used are shown in Fig. 1. Full details of the kinetic rationale used in designing this combination have been provided previously (Price and Hill 1977; Price et al. 1983).

The protocol required that the standard medical precautions listed in Table 1 were observed in all patients. The therapeutic strategy was to give the first course of schedule A chemotherapy on day 1 and the second course on day 14 and to assess response to this initial chemotherapy on day 28. Local "curative" therapy with radiotherapy and/or salvage surgery was started on day 28 and the overall final response was assessed 4-6 weeks after its completion. A response (partial) was defined as a reduction of at least 50% in the product of two perpendicular diameters of all measurable lesions. A complete remission (CR) was defined as the absence of clinically detectable disease. Response rates were compared using the chi-squared test with Yates' correction. *P*-values were determined by the two-tailed test. Survival was calculated by a life table method and compared using a log rank test.

Results

Response to Chemotherapy

One hundred and sixty-seven patients were assessed for response to two courses of initial schedule A chemotherapy on day 28. Reasons for nonassessment in eight patients were as follows: tumor measurements inadequate, five; surgical intervention within 6 days of the first course of chemotherapy, two; treatment-related death involving a protocol violation (discussed below), one. One hundred and thirty patients were male and 37 female, with an age range of 30-80 years (median 57 years). One hundred and eight patients (65%) had an objective response to chemotherapy and 59 (35%) were classed as nonresponders, although 16 had a minimal 20% -30% response. The response rate to initial chemotherapy was higher in the 96 patients with stage III disease than in the 71 patients with stage IV disease (70% versus 58% respectively). Chemotherapy response was not significantly influenced by sex or histological tumor grade. However, as shown in Table 2, site and age were important predictive factors for response. The response rates for oral cavity and nasopharyngeal lesions were significantly better than those for all other sites ($P<0.05$ and $P<0.01$ respectively), while hypopharyngeal tumors responded poorly compared with all other sites ($P<0.1$). Patients aged 49 years or less were more likely to respond to chemotherapy than older patients ($P<0.01$).

Response to Local Therapies

Response to local therapy after chemotherapy was assessed in 167 patients. Details of the local therapies recieved were as follows: 63% of patients had radiation only, 32% had radiation plus surgery, and 5% had surgery only. An overall final CR rate of 63% was achieved with results by stage being 74% and 49% for stage III and IV disease respectively.

Table 2. Factors influencing the response rate to chemotherapy

	Chemotherapy responders/nonresponders		
	Overall (%)	Stage III (%)	Stage IV (%)
Analysis by age:			
≦49 years	37/ 8 (82%)[a]	21/ 3 (88%)[b]	16/ 5 (76%)[a]
>49 years	69/53 (57%)[a]	43/27 (61%)[b]	26/26 (50%)[a]
Analysis by site:			
Oral cavity	29/ 8 (78%)	22/ 6	7/ 2
Oropharynx	19/15 (56%)	10/ 2	6/13
Nasopharynx	18/ 3 (86%)	6/ 1	12/ 2
Hypopharynx	12/11 (52%)	7/ 6	5/ 5
Larynx:			
Supraglottic	16/12	8/ 6	8/ 6
Glottic	12/ 9	11/ 7	1/ 2
Subglottic	1/ 0	1/ 0	0/ 0
Others	4/ 2	2/ 1	2/ 1

[a] $P<0.01$; [b] $P<0.05$

Table 3. Incidence of side effects from 370 cycles of schedule A chemotherapy given to 175 eligible patients

Side effect	No. of cycles	No. of patients
Myelosuppression ($WBC < 3000/mm^3$)	7 (2%)	5 (3%)
Mucositis (mild - no intubation)	26 (7%)	18 (10%)
Nephrotoxicity	0	0
Peripheral neuropathy	10 (3%)	8 (5%)
Pulmonary (chest pains)	1	1
Skin rash	24 (6%)	14 (8%)
Alopecia	12 (3%)	10 (6%)
Nausea and vomiting	20 (5%)	14 (8%)
Anorexia	5 (1%)	3 (2%)
Malaise and lethargy	12 (3%)	6 (3%)
Deaths (protocol violations)	2	2

Table 4. Median durations of survival in months: analysis by stage

	Stage III	Stage IV
All eligible patients	37.5[c]	16.6[c]
Chemotherapy responders	38.0	22.0[b]
Chemotherapy nonresponders	18.4	8.4[b]
Patients in final CR after local therapy	96+[a]	63.6[a]
Patients with RD at final assessment	8.3[a]	7.7[a]

[a] $P < 0.00005$; [b] P, 0.008; [c] P, 0.02

For all patients as a group this final CR rate was significantly greater in chemotherapy responders (76%) than in chemotherapy nonresponders (39%) ($P < 0.001$). Analyses by stage showed improved CR figures for chemotherapy responders (8%) versus nonresponders (60%) in stage III disease and highly significant benefit in stage IV disease with figures of 69% for chemotherapy responders versus 23% for nonresponders ($P < 0.001$).

Toxicity

Toxicity associated with schedule A chemotherapy was minimal and there was 100% patient compliance. The side effects observed in this study are summarized in Table 3. They necessitated no change of chemotherapy dosage or timing except for one patient who developed a severe skin reaction and bleomycin was omitted from the second chemotherapy course. Myelosuppression was negligible, with only one patient having a white cell count (WBC) nadir below $2000/mm^3$. This patient had known impaired renal function (creati-

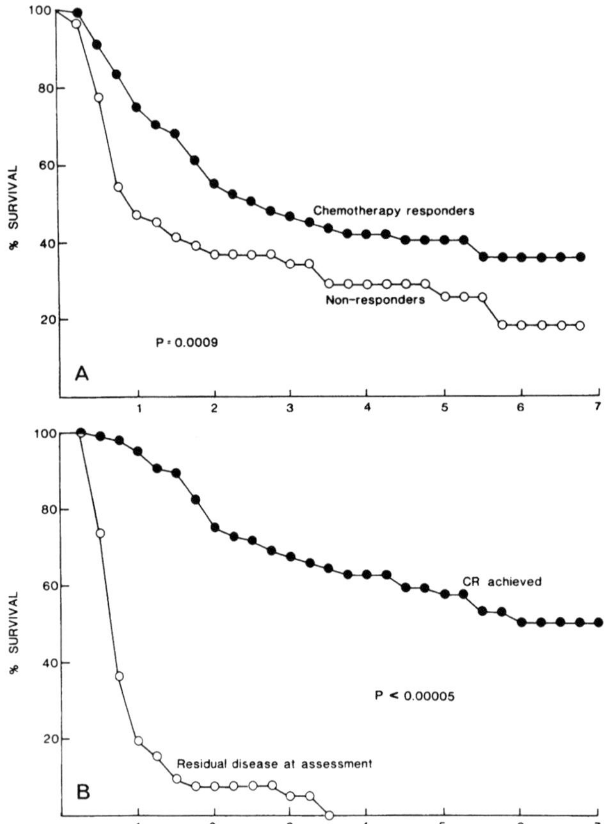

Fig. 2 A, B. Actuarial survival data: **A** Influence of initial response to schedule A chemotherapy on survival. **B** Influence of overall final response after chemotherapy *and* local therapy on survival

nine clearance <70 ml/min) and the stated medical precautions were not observed, since a prolonged folinic acid "rescue" was not administered, and died from the treatment. The second death also resulted from a protocol violation since the second course of chemotherapy was administered when the patient's white cell count was $3000/mm^3$ whereas the normal level was $10000/mm^3$.

Survival

Overall survival data for the 175 eligible patients are available, with a median follow-up of 66 months. These are summarized in Table 4 and Fig. 2. All patients with stage III disease had a median survival of 37.5 months. The figure for patients with stage IV disease was significantly lower at 16.6 months (P, 0.02). Overall chemotherapy responders lived significantly longer than nonresponders (P, 0.0009), as shown in Fig. 2 A. Response to initial schedule A chemotherapy was therefore a good prognostic sign. By stage (see Table 4), this difference was statistically significant only in stage IV disease (P, 0.008).

The importance of achieving a final CR was emphasized by these data. All patients achieving a CR after local therapy lived significantly longer than those with residual disease (RD) at assessment ($P<0.00005$, see Fig. 2 B). This difference was significant

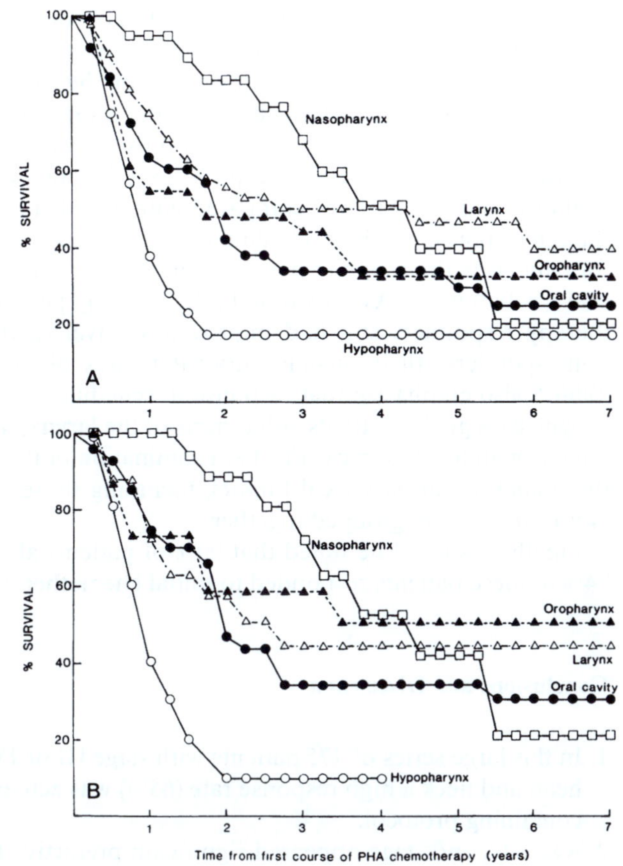

Fig. 3 A, B. Actuarial survival data: **A** Analysis of 175 eligible patients by tumor site. **B** Analysis of initial chemotherapy responders only by tumor site

Table 5. Median durations of survival in months: analysis by site of all patients

Site	All patients	Chemotherapy responders	Chemotherapy nonresponders	Patients achieving a final CR
Nasopharynx	44.9	51.7	12+	52.5
Oropharynx	20.1	50+	8.7	96+
Oral cavity	22.4	23.5	6.0	57.1
Hypopharynx	10.1	10.6	8.3	96+
Larynx	51.2	30.4	50+	84+
Overall *P* values	0.0002	0.007	0.016	NS

($P<0.00005$) irrespective of stage (see Table 4). Improved survival figures (data not shown) were also noted in those patients achieving a final CR who were aged 49 years or less compared with the older patient group.

Analysis by site (see Fig. 3, Table 5) showed that for all patients (Fig. 3 A) those with nasopharyngeal and laryngeal tumors had the best survival figures, while patients with hypopharyngeal, oropharyngeal, or oral cavity lesions had the poorest survival figures (*P*, 0.0002 for the overall group). For chemotherapy responders only (see Fig. 3 B), patients with nasopharyngeal and oropharyngeal tumors did well compared with tumors at all other sites. The survival figures for patients with nasopharyngeal tumors were statistically significantly better than those with tumors of the oral cavity (*P*, 0.01), hypopharynx (*P*, 0.0001), and larynx (*P*, 0.05). For oropharyngeal tumors, however, the survival figures were significantly different only from those of the hypopharynx (*P*, 0.06). Since the response rate to initial chemotherapy was significantly higher in patients with nasopharyngeal or oral cavity tumors, compared with all other sites (see Table 2), it follows that although response to initial schedule A chemotherapy was a very favorable prognostic sign for patients with nasopharyngeal tumors, this was, unexpectedly, far less so for those with oral cavity tumors. As shown in Table 5, among patients with oral cavity tumors chemotherapy responders still had improved survival figures compared with chemotherapy nonresponders; their median survival figures of only 24 months were poor. Date in Table 5 also emphasize that response to schedule A chemotherapy appeared an adverse prognostic sign for patients eith tumors of the larynx, *unless* they went on the achieve a final CR with local therapy. Further examination of these data is now under way since for these analyses all laryngeal tumors, including those of the supraglottic, subglottic, and glottic areas, were grouped together.

Finally, it should be noted that 90% of patients alive at 6 years were disease free and 74% of these patients responded to initial chemotherapy.

Conclusions and Discussion

1. In this large series of 175 patients with stage III or IV squamous cell carcinomas of the head and neck a high response rate (65%) was achieved safely using this non-cisplatin-containing protocol.
2. Age, site, and stage appeared significant predictive factors for response to schedule A chemotherapy.
3. Schedule A chemotherapy did not compromise subsequent radiation therapy: 80% of all patients were given full-dose uninterrupted radiotherapy.
4. Chemotherapy responders lived significantly longer than chemotherapy nonresponders, (*P*, 0.00009 for all patients): by stage this difference was highly significant statistically for stage IV disease (*P*, 0.008)
5. Significantly more chemotherapy responders achieved a complete remission than nonresponders ($P < 0.001$ for all patients): by stage this difference was highly significant statistically for stage IV disease ($P < 0.001$)
6. Achievement of complete remission increased survival very significantly, irrespective of disease stage
7. Response to initial schedule A chemotherapy was a favorable prognostic sign for patients with nasopharyngeal tumors, less so for those with oral cavity lesions and apparently *not* for those with laryngeal tumors.

This study was closed in January 1984. These patients will now be followed up so as to provide 10-year survival data, including detailed site by site analyses.

One of the major advantages of this schedule A chemotherapy protocol is its lack of toxicity compared with a number of other currently used cisplatin-containing schedules (see Table 6). However, it should be emphasized that this safety is achieved without loss of therapeutic effect since the 65% response rate noted in this large series of 175 patients is comparable with the 70%–80% figures quoted by other workers in small groups of pat-

Table 6. Summary of toxicities from some recent studies using cisplatin-containing drug combinations compared with Price-Hill schedula A chemotherapy

Drugs used	Days on treatment per course	Nausea and vomiting	Significant myelotoxicity	Renal toxicity	Reference
CDDP+VCR +BLM	5	71%	27%	10%	Al Sarraf et al. (1981)
CDDP+BLM	9	Moderate	2%	9%	Hong et al. (1981)
CDDP+BLM	9	100%	5%	20%	Pennachio et al. (1982)
CDDP+VCR +BLM	7	100%	2%	19%	Spaulding et al. (1982)
CDDP+5FU	6	64%	39%	33%	Kish et al. (1982)
CDDP+BLM +VBL	9	100%	5%	3% Severe	Davis et al. (1983)
CDDP+BLM +VBL+MTX +5FU	4	100%	36%	68%	Krasnow et al. (1984)
CDDP+BLM	8	75%	8% Severe	1% Severe	Wolf et al. (1984)
VCR+BLM+ MTX+5FU	2	8%	3%	0%	Personal results

CDDP, cisplatin; *VCR*, vincristine; *BLM*, bleomycin; *5FU*, 5-fluorouracil; *VLB*, vinblastine; *MTX*, methotrexate

ients, frequently numbering less than 50 (see Table 7). However, our quoted complete response rate to initial schedule A chemotherapy is low, but this figure of 7% does not provide a fair assessment of the efficacy of schedule A alone since response was assessed on day 28 after only two courses of chemotherapy after which patients were started on radiation therapy even while their tumors were still regressing from the drug treatment. Considerable interest has been raised recently in the very high complete response rates of approximately 54% achieved following three courses of initial chemotherapy consisting of cisplatin plus a 5-fluorouracil infusion (Kish et al. 1984). These are very impressive figures, which it is hoped will translate into prolonged, good-quality survival. However, while it has been reported recently that survival figures are superior in those patients who achieved a complete response with the cisplatin-fluorouracil combination alone compared with those requiring both chemotherapy and radiotherapy to reach a CR, the median survival figures quoted of 72 and 46 weeks respectively are disappointing (Ensley et al. 1984). Neither of these figures appear as promising as the median survival data quoted here from our study or that of Hong et al. (1984) (see Table 7). In addition, while we are able to provide long-term follow-up data from our series, as indicated in Table 7, this is not the case yet for most of the studies using cisplatin-containing combinations. Long-term follow-up is essential before definitive answers can be provided as to whether or not cisplatin should automatically be included in adjuvant chemotherapy for head and neck tumors.

This present study also provides the first very important demonstration that initial chemotherapy may be valuable in treating only tumors at certain sites within the head and

Table 7. Comparative response rates and survival figures from recent studies using cisplatin-containing drug combinations compared with Price-Hill schedule A chemotherapy

Drugs used	No. of cycles	No. of patients	Response to chemotherapy		% NED after all therapies	Survival data	Reference
			CR	CR+PR			
CDDP+VCR +BLM	2	77	29%	80%	NS	At 18 months: 46% alive, 29% NED CR to chemotherapy - 55% alive PR to chemotherapy - 38% alive	Al Sarraf et al. (1981)
CDDP+BLM	1/2	41	17%	70%	73%	At 20 months: 53% alive, 41% NED	Pennachio et al. (1982)
CDDP+VCR +BLM	2	48	23%	88%	40%	At 27 months: 40% NED (median)	Spaulding et al. (1982)
CDDP+BLM +VLB	≦4	64	22%	44%	84% control of local disease	Median survivals (months): CR to chemotherapy - 52 PR to chemotherapy - 12 At 5 years only 17% NED	Davis et al. (1983) Perry et al. (1984)
CDDP+VLB +5FU	2	27	4%	80%	56%	At 10 months: 60% NED	Spaulding et al. (1983)
CDDP+BLM	1/2	61	20%	73%	75%	Median survivals (months): Final CRs - 36+ CR to chemotherapy - 58 PR to chemotherapy - 26	Hong et al. (1984)
CDDP+5FU	2 3	26 85	19% 54%	88% 93%	NS NS	Median survivals (months): After 2 courses - 13 After 3 courses - 18+ (28% alive at 18m)	Kish et al. (1984)
CDDP+BLM +VLB+MTX +5FU	3	25	36%	68%	48%	At 9-19 months: CR to chemotherapy 77% NED; PR to chemotherapy - 66% NED	Krasnow et al. (1984)
VCR+BLM+ MTX+5FU	2	175	7%	65%	63%	Median survivals (months): Final CRs - 96+ PR to chemotherapy - 31 At 5 years 35% NED	Price and Hill (1985)

NED, no clinical evidence of disease; *CR*, complete response; *PR*, partial response; *CDDP*, cisplatin; *VCR*, vincristine; *BLM*, bleomycin; *VLB*, vinblastine; *5FU*, 5-fluorouracil; *MTX*, methotrexate

neck region. We suggest therefore that squamous cell carcinomas of the head and neck should no longer be grouped as if they were one disease entity but that randomized, prospective, controlled clinical trials should be carried out using initial chemotherapy to see which sites will benefit in terms of increased good-quality survival.

Finally, the need remains for definitive results from randomized, prospective controlled clinical studies to determine the impact of this combined modality therapy, using initial chemotherapy on overall survival. While preliminary results from a few such studies are not encouraging, they do show that single-agent methotrexate (Taylor et al. 1984) or a single course of an initial cisplatin combination (Jacobs et al. 1984) are inadequate. However, rather than inferring from this work that all chemotherapy is ineffective, the challenge remains to establish the value of initial full-dose intensive combination chemotherapy in advanced head and neck cancer, since it seems at present highly probable that cure rates can be increased at certain sites with significantly less mutilation, using treatments and concepts available now.

Acknowledgments. We are particularly indebted to Mr. Henry Shaw and Dr. Vera Dalley for referring patients into this study at the Royal Marsden, to Dr. Eileen Busby for providing details of the radiotherapy administered, and to Dr. Ken MacRae for his statistical expertise. We are grateful to Alison Barrow for her secretarial assistance.

References

Al-Sarraf M, Drelichman A, Jacobs J, Kinzie J, Hoschner J, Loh J, Weaver A (1981) Adjuvant chemotherapy with cis-platinum, oncovin, and bleomycin followed by surgery and/or radiotherapy in patients with advanced previously untreated head and neck cancer: final report. In: Salmon SE, Jones SE (eds) Adjuvant therapy of cancer III. Grune and Stratton, New York, pp 145-152

Davis KR, Perry DJ, Zajtchuk JT (1983) Induction chemotherapy with vinblastine, bleomycin and cis-diamminedichloroplatinum in squamous cell carcinoma of the head and neck. Otolaryngol Head Neck Surg 91: 627-631

DeVita VT (1984) Opening comments: Only if you believe in magic. In: Jones SE, Salmon SE (eds) Adjuvant therapy of cancer IV. Grune and Stratton, Orlando, pp 3-16

Ensley J, Kish J, Jacobs J, Weaver A, Crissman J, Kinzie J, Al-Sarraf M, Vaitkevicius V (1984) Superior survival in complete responders achieved with chemotherapy alone compared to those requiring chemotherapy and radiotherapy in patients with advanced squamous cell cancer of the head and neck. Proc ASCO 3: 181 (Abstract C-704)

Hill BT, Price LA, Busby E, MacRae K, Shaw JH (1984) Positive impact of initial 24-hour combination chemotherapy without cis-platinum on 6-year survival figures in advanced squamous cell carcinomas of the head and neck. In: Jones SE, Salmon SE (eds) Adjuvant therapy of cancer IV. Grune and Stratton, Orlando, pp 97-106

Hong WK, Pennachio J, Shapsay S, Vaughan C, Katz A, Bhutani R, Bromer R, Willett B, Strong S (1981) Adjuvant chemotherapy with cis-platinum and bleomycin infusion prior to definitive treatment for advanced stage III and IV squamous cell head and neck carcinoma. In: Salmon SE, Jones SE (eds) Adjuvant therapy of cancer III. Grune and Stratton, New York, pp 153-160

Hong WK, Popkin J, Bromer R, Shapsay S, Hoffer S, Willett B, Strong MS, Vaughan C, Katz A, Fofonoff S, Amato D (1984) Adjuvant chemotherapy as initial treatment of advanced head and neck cancer: survival data at three years. In: Jones SE, Salmon SE (eds) Adjuvant therapy of cancer IV. Grune and Stratton, Orlando, pp 127-133

Jacobs C, Wolf GT, Mekuch RW, Vikram B (1984) Adjuvant chemotherapy for head and neck squamous carcinomas. Proc ASCO 4: 182 (Abstract C-708)

Kish J, Drelichman A, Jacobs J, Hoschner J, Kinzie J, Loh J, Weaver A, Al-Sarraf M (1982) Clinical trial of cisplatin and 5-FU infusion as initial treatment for advanced squamous cell carcinoma of the head and neck. Cancer Treat Rep 66: 471-474

Kish JA, Ensley J, Weaver A, Jacobs JR, Kinzie J, Cummings G, Al-Sarraf M (1984) Improvement of complete response rate to induction adjuvant chemotherapy for advanced squamous carcinoma of the head and neck. In: Jones SE, Salmon SE (eds) Adjuvant therapy of cancer IV. Grune and Stratton, Orlando, pp 107-115

Krasnow SH, Cohen MH, Johnston-Early A, Citron ML, Fossieck BE, Mauk CM, Yenson A, Banda FP, Lunzer S, deFries HO (1984) Combined therapy for Stage III-IV head and neck cancer: preliminary results. J Clin Oncol 2: 804-810

Pennachio JL, Hong WK, Shapsay S, Gillis T, Vaughan C, Bhutani R, Ucmakli A, Katz AE, Bromer R, Willett B, Strong SM (1982) Combination of cis-platinum and bleomycin prior to surgery and/

or radiotherapy compared with radiotherapy alone for the treatment of advanced squamous cell carcinoma of the head and neck. Cancer 50: 2795-2801
Perry DJ, Davis RK, Zajtchuk JR, Baumann JC (1984) Bleomycin and cisplatin in the treatment of squamous carcinoma of the head and neck. In: Jones SE, Salmon SE (eds) Adjuvant therapy of cancer IV. Grune and Stratton, Orlando, pp 135-143
Price LA, Hill BT (1977) A kinetically-based logical approach to the chemotherapy of head and neck cancer. Clin Otolaryngol 2: 339-345
Price LA, Hill BT (1982) Safe and effective induction chemotherapy without cisplatin for squamous cell carcinoma of the head and neck: impact on complete response rate and survival at five years, following local therapy. Med Ped Oncol 10: 535-548
Price LA, Hill BT, Calvert AH, Shaw JH, Hughes KB (1975) Kinetically-based multiple drug treatment for advanced head and neck cancer. Br Med J 3: 10-11
Price LA, MacRae K, Hill BT (1983) Integration of safe initial combination chemotherapy (without cisplatin) with a high response rate and local therapy for untreated stage III and IV epidermoid cancer of the head and neck: 5-year survival data. Cancer Treat Rep 67: 535-539
Spaulding MB, Kahn A, De Los Santos R, Klotch D, Lore JM (1982) Adjuvant chemotherapy in advanced head and neck cancer. Am J Surg 144: 432-436
Spaulding MB, Vasquez J, Khan A, Sundquist N, Lore JM (1983) A nontoxic treatment for advanced head and neck cancer. Arch Otolaryngol 109: 789-791
Taylor SG, Caldarelli DD, Norusis M, Showell JL, Hutchinson JC, Holinger LD, Murthy AK, Applebaum E (1984) A randomized trial of adjuvant chemotherapy in head and neck squamous cancer. In: Jones SE, Salmon SE (eds) Adjuvant therapy of cancer IV. Grune and Stratton, Orlando, pp 89-96
Wolf GT, Makuch RW, Baker SR (1984) Predictive factors for tumor response to preoperative chemotherapy in patients with head and neck squamous carcinoma. Cancer 54: 2869-2877

Chemotherapy with or Without Anticoagulation as Initial Management of Patients with Operable Colorectal Cancer: A Prospective Study with at Least 5 Years Follow-up

A. N. Papaioannou, A. P. Polychronis, J. A. Kozonis, J. Nomicos, M. Tsamouri, G. A. Plataniotis, and J. K. Papageorgiou

Department of Surgery, Mount Vernon Hospital, 12 North Seventh Avenue, Mount Vernon, NY 10550, USA

Colorectal carcinoma (CRCa) is the most frequently encountered malignant neoplasm in the United States, which ultimately kills almost exclusively because of systemic dissemination in more than 50% of those manifesting the disease (Welch and Donaldson 1974). It is obvious that better means for systemic control of this disease are needed. The design of this study was influenced by (a) dissatisfaction with the results of postoperative adjuvant chemotherapy in CRCa, (b) the many theoretical considerations along with some experimental and clinical studies suggesting that chemotherapy might become more effective if given before operation rather than after it, and (c) evidence suggesting that anticoagulation might hinder tumor growth. This study was recently reported in detail (Papaioannou et al. 1985) and is presented here in shortened form.

Patients, Methods, and Results

All patients admitted to the B Surgical Unit of the Evangelismos Hospital, Athens, with histologically proven or strongly suspected carcinoma of the colon or rectum by clinical history, physical examination, and endoscopic and/or radiologic criteria were considered for this study. Anemic patients were transfused to hematocrit 40% prior to chemotherapy or surgery. Preoperative workup included liver scan, alkaline phosphatase, and αGT in addition to routine investigations and barium enema. Other investigations on the basis of individual patient's symptoms were also carried out. Excluded were patients whose cardiac status precluded long-term administration of Adriamycin, those whose work-up was highly suggestive of metastatic disease in the liver or other organs, those who were found to have metastatic liver disease or peritoneal implants at operation, and finally those with history of another treated malignant neoplasm other than in the skin. Also excluded were patients 76 years or older. The study was instituted in November 1976 and was closed at the end of 1979. This trial was initially set up as two separate studies: the first to test the value of preoperative chemotherapy (PrCh) with controls receiving postoperative chemotherapy alone and the second to test the combination of PrCh plus heparin anticoagulation, compared with postoperative chemotherapy alone. As the accrual of patients was slow, the two control groups were unified and the two studies became one with three arms. This has created the discrepancy of numbers between patients of the control and each of the two other arms. Thus, the three arms were as follows:

Group I: One cycle of PrCH + operation with intraoperative chemotherapy + 11 cycles of postoperative chemotherapy

Recent Results in Cancer Research. Vol 103

Group II: One cycle of PrCh + heparin + operation with intraoperative chemotherapy + 11 cycles of postoperative chemotherapy
Group III: No PrCh, operation + 12 cycles of postoperative chemotherapy

The preoperative cycle consisted of day 1, vincristine 2 mg; day 2, Adriamycin 40 mg and 5-fluorouracil 500 mg; day 3, 5-fluorouracil 500 mg; day 4, 5-fluorouracil 500 mg and Adriamycin 40 mg.

Intraoperative chemotherapy consisted of 5-fluorouracil 1000 mg in 1000 ml 5% dextrose in water i. v. drip, beginning ½ h prior to exploration. The infusion was continued throughout the entire duration of operation and for about 6 h.

All postoperative cycles consisted of *day 1,* vincristine 2 mg; day 2, 5-fluorouracil 1000 mg and Adriamycin 40 mg i. v., and *days 1–5;* cyclophosphamide 150 mg daily by mouth.

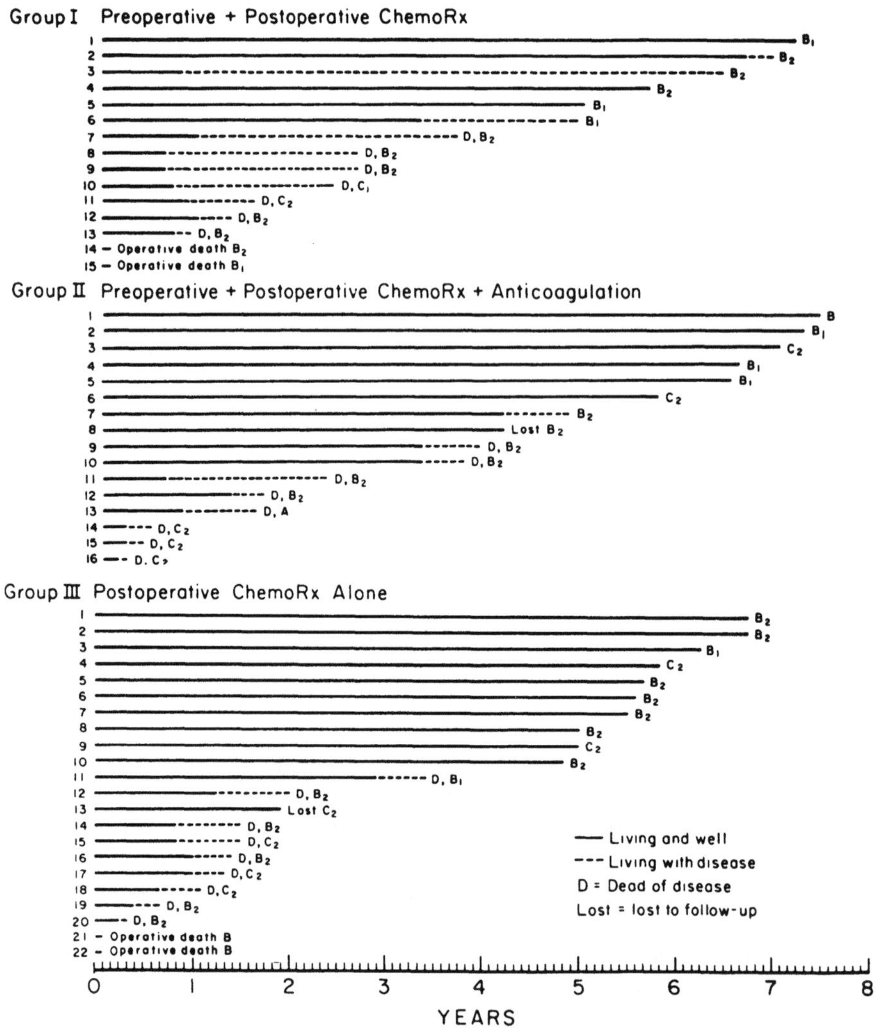

Fig. 1. Patient disease-free interval, survival, and pathological stage by treatment category. *chemoRx,* chemotherapy

Table 1. Survival of patients with Recurrence (Months)

Group	Surgery to recurrence	Recurrence to death		Surgery to death	
		Mean	Significance	Mean	Significance
I	19.8	20.4	I vs. III $P<0.05$	40.2	I vs. III $P<0.05$
II	19.1	6.5	II vs. III NS	25.7	II vs. III $P<0.1$
I and II	19.5	13.8	I and II vs. III $P<0.1$	33.3	I and II vs. III $P<0.05$
III	12.2	5.4		17.7	

NS, not significant

Heparin was given as a continuous i.v. drip containing 12500 units sodium heparin in 500 ml saline, which was renewed every 12 h for a daily dose of about 25000 units/day per patient, to maintain clotting time beyond 30 min. Anticoagulation was given 1 day before, during, and 1 day after this chemotherapy cycle.

The three groups had a comparable distribution of abdominal perineal resections and colectomies, and of postoperative complications, but a slightly older mean age in group III. As far as the stage of disease was concerned, the three groups were not entirely comparable but the differences were not substantial. This is further discussed below.

Measurable differences in tumor size following PrCh where this could be adequately evaluated, e.g., in the rectum, were not observed. However, as a rule, the tumor 2 weeks before PrCh would look less bloody and friable and in some instances a better mobility of its base could be appreciated on palpation. Likewise, when histological sections from biopsy specimens before PrCh were compared with those from the resected specimens after one cycle of PrCh, no distinct histological changes could be identified in the morphology of the tumor. However, when all patients in each group were considered together, some minor differences could be appreciated between the three groups, e.g., in the degree of necrosis and ulceration present (less in the two groups receiving PrCh) and of fibrosis present (higher in group III).

Survival duration and the pathological stage distribution of each patient are shown in Fig. 1. Substantial differences in survival are not seen among the three groups. However, if only the cases that developed recurrences are considered, all deaths but one in the control group occurred within 2 years from operation, whereas only one-half of those occurring in the groups receiving PrCh took place before the end of the 2nd postoperative year. Compared with group III, patients in group I and II who ultimately developed recurrence, had a longer period of recurrence-free interval as well as longer survival from surgery to death. These differences were statistically significant (see Table 1).

Discussion

The value of PrCh and the various arguments in support of this principle are discussed in the paper on gastric cancer (Papaioannou et al., this volume). All arguments discussed with respect to PrCh in gastric cancer apply to colorectal carcinoma as well. Insofar as the choice of chemotherapeutic regimen is concerned, despite experimental evidence suggesting that single agents would be effective if used when the tumor burden is low (Schabel 1975), meaningful differences were not observed in any of the early large-scale trials using single agents (Dwight et al. 1973; Dixon et al. 1971; Higgins et al. 1978; Grage et al. 1979). Only in one trial (Grage et al. 1979) did Dukes C patients with rectal cancer have a statistically significant increase noted in the disease-free interval and in survival. Conversely, interest had been increasing in the many theoretical advantages of combination chemotherapy and there were some encouraging reports. It was, therefore, decided to combine most agents known to have some activity in advanced disease. The nitrosoureas were not included because they are highly immunosuppressive and their use in the preoperative regimen would have precluded operation for at least 6 weeks.

Anticoagulation has been repeatedly in the treatment of cancer used in the past (for reviews see Hilgard and Thornes 1976; Hoover and Ketcham 1975; Zacharski et al. 1979).

For example, agents which will interfere in some way with the formation of clot have an antitumor effect. This has been shown experimentally with heparin (Agostino and Cliffton 1963), warfarin, urokinase and streptokinase (Thornes 1974), aspirin (Gasic et al. 1972), dextran (Suemasu 1970), dipyridamole and its derivatives (Ambrus et al. 1975), and agents inducing hypofibrinogenemia (Williams and Maugham 1972). Conversely, conditions which enhance coagulation will increase the incidence of experimental metastases, e.g., epsilon-aminocaproic acid, induction of hyperfibrinogenemia, activation of factor XII (Agostino 1970), and administration of endotoxin, which stimulates tissue factor activation in leukocytes (Lerner et al. 1971). Fibrinogen is taken up by many types of malignancy and its reduction is associated with a more favorable tumor course (Schaffer 1964). In general, the tumor inhibition observed with anticoagulation may be due to either a direct effect of coagulation inhibition upon tumor growth or to potentiation of host resistance mechanisms. The formation of clot at the periphery of the tumor may enhance tumor growth by facilitating attachments of tumor cells to the endothelium, by providing nutrients or growth stimulants, or by serving as a structural lattice for tumor proliferation. Alternatively, the clot may provide protection against host defense mechanisms (Hilgard and Thornes 1976). Likewise, the anticoagulant may have a direct stimulatory effect on resistance effector cells (Hilgard and Thornes 1976; Schultz et al. 1977).

In man several studies have shown that anticoagulants can affect the natural history of tumors as well as patient survival. Thornes, for example (Thornes 1974), showed that the need for chemotherapeutic agents in controlling the disease decreased when warfarin was added. Patients with advanced malignancies given warfarin in addition to chemotherapy had a 40.6% 2-year survival, contrasted to a 17.8% survival for the control group who were treated by chemotherapy alone. Other patients with a variety of tumors in different primary sites benefited by anticoagulants or fibrinolytic agents, e.g., ovary, breasts, lymphoma and leukemia (Thornes 1972), promyelocytic leukemia (Drapkin et al. 1978), and squamous cell carcinoma of the lung (Elias et al. 1975). It is particularly interesting that regression was possible in some of these tumors even if they were highly resistant to chemotherapy. Likewise, another study indicated some benefit by treatment with warfarin of patients with pancreatic carcinoma (Waddell 1973) and with stage II and III carcinoma of the uterine cervix (Ries et al. 1968), and in patients with cancer of the breast, lung, and colon treated by defibrination (Williams and Maugham 1972). Likewise, Hoover et al. (1978) using warfarin as an adjuvant to amputation for osteosarcoma showed a distinct survival advantage of the treated patients. Another line of evidence comes from prospective large-scale studies of patients receiving anticoagulants prophylactically against cardiovascular disease. The incidence of malignancy in the patients treated was considerably lower than that of their counterparts serving as controls (Michaels 1974). Some workers

Table 2. Disease stage distribution (Dukes)

Stage	Frequency distribution				
	Astler-Coller I and II (%)			III	
		(#)	(%)	(#)	(%)
A	0.3	1	3.2	-	0
B_1	13.6	7	22.5	2	9.0
B_2	46.6	16	51.6	14	63.6
C_1	4.0	1	3.2	-	0
C_2	35.5	6	19.3	6	27.1
B_2+C	86.1	23	74.1	20	90.7

observed no benefit from anticoagulation (Edlis et al. 1976; Rohwedder and Sagastume 1977) but to our knowledge acceleration of tumor growth has never been observed.

We elected to use heparin rather than other anticoagulants mainly influenced by work demonstrating that the tumoricidal function of macrophages was enhanced by heparin most likely through interferon production (Schultz et al. 1977). Heparin is also easy to administer and counteract and it becomes immediately effective. Hopefully, the sludging and the slow and inefficient circulation existing in the center of tumors might be overcome by heparin, thus enhancing delivery as well as efficacy of concomitantly administered chemotherapy. For all the above reasons, we used full anticoagulation 1 day before, during, and for 1 day following the completion of the chemotherapy cycle.

With the small numbers of evaluable patients available in this study, we are unable to conclude either that PrCh is truly effective or that it is an ineffective means to deal with CRCa. This is particularly so in view of an apparently ineffective chemotherapeutic regimen, as suggested by the lack of substantial size reduction of the primaries and the absence of any impact on survival. The increase of the free interval from surgery to recurrence as well as the survival from recurrence to death as it was significantly and consistently observed for both groups receiving PrCh is encouraging (Table 1). It is possible that PrCh is more effective than chemotherapy given postoperatively because it affects primarily micrometastases which are presumably more vulnerable to PrCh (Schabel 1975; Papaioannou 1981). The lower incidence of combined Dukes B2 and C pathological lesions in groups 1 and 2 compared with group 3 as well as compared with other series not receiving any therapy suggests that the tumors as a group were in fact downstaged (Table 2). Could PrCh have had more impressive effects had it been continued for two to three cycles? Interruption of its beneficial impact on the natural history of the tumor may have accounted for the course of events seen in our study. Currently the NSABP is repeating an encouraging study showing the most impressive results to date on long-term survival in patients with CRCa (Taylor 1981). This was accomplished through a short course of 5-fluorouracil plus heparin delivered through a portal catheter for 7 days after operation, starting on the day of colectomy. Whether or not the timing rather than the route of administration is the important feature here remains to be investigated. One factor, however, that should be taken into account is the possible antitumor effects of intraportal administration of heparin. If the observations of Schultz et al (1977) are applicable to human macrophages, the intraportal administration of heparin may well have important antitumor properties, not only by interfering with clotting but also, as a continuous stimulant of the resident macrophages in the liver, by rendering them tumoricidal.

In our study, the addition of heparin in the single preoperative chemotherapy cycle had no appreciable influence on survival. This, however, does not mean that the principle itself is in error. No impact on the survival of the percentage of surviving patients could be documented. Further study of both PrCh and of anticoagulation appears to be justified particularly as more effective agents become available for this disease.

References

Agostino D (1970) Enhancement of pulmonary metastasis following intravenous infusion of a suspension of ellagic acid. Tumori 56: 29-35

Agostino D, Cliffton EE (1973) Decrease in pulmonary metastases: potentiation of nitrogen mustard effect by heparin and fibrinolysin. Ann Surg 157: 400-408

Ambrus JL, Ambrus CM, Pickern J, Solder S, Bross I (1975) Hematologic changes and thromboembolic complications in neoplastic disease and their relationship to metastasis. J Med 6: 433-458

Dixon JW, Longmire WP, Holden WD (1971) The use of triethylene triophosphamide: an adjuvant to surgical treatment of gastric and colorectal cancer: ten-year follow-up. Ann Surg 173: 26-39

Drapkin RL, Gee TS, Dowling MD, Arlin Z, McKenzie S, Kempin S, Clarkson B (1978) Prophylactic heparin therapy in acute promyelocytic leukemia. Cancer 41: 2484-2490

Dwight RW, Humphrey EW, Higgins GA, et al. (1973) FUDR, an adjuvant to surgery of the large bowel. J Surg Oncol 5: 243-249

Edlis HE, Goudsmit A, Brindley C, Niemetz J (1976) Trial of heparin and cyclophosphamide (NSC-26271) in the treatment of lung cancer. Cancer Treat Rep 60: 575-578

Elias EG, Shulka SK, Mink I (1975) Heparin and chemotherapy in the management of inoperable lung cancer. Cancer 36: 129-136

Gasic GJ, Gasic TB, Murphy S (1972) Antimetastatic effect of aspirin. Lancet 2: 932

Grage T, Hill G, Cornell T, et al. (1979) Adjuvant chemotherapy in large bowel cancer: updated analysis of single-agent chemotherapy. In: Jones SE, Salmon SE (eds) Adjuvant therapy of cancer II. Grune and Stratton, New York

Higgins GA, Lee LE, Dwight RW, Keehn RJ (1978) The case of adjuvant 5-fluorouracil in colorectal cancer. Cancer Clin Trials 1: 35-41

Hilgard P, Thornes RD (1976) Anticoagulants in the treatment of cancer. Eur J Cancer 12: 755-762

Hoover HC, Ketcham AS (1975) Decreasing experimental metastasis formation with anticoagulation and chemotherapy. Surg Forum 26: 173-174

Hoover HC Jr, Ketcham AS, Millar RC, et al (1978) Osteosarcoma: improved survival with anticoagulation and amputation. Cancer 41: 2475-2480

Lerner RG, Goldstein R, Cummings G (1971) Stimulation of human leukocyte thromboplastic activity by endotoxin. Proc Soc Exp Biol Med 138: 145-148

Michaels L (1974) The incidence and course of cancer in patients receiving anticoagulant therapy. J Med 5: 98-106

Papaioannou AN (1981) Perspectives in cancer research: preoperative chemotherapy for operable solid tumors. Eur J Cancer 17: 963-969

Papaioannou AN, Polychronis A, Plataniotis G, Tsamouri M, Kozonis J, Nomicos J (1985) Chemotherapy as initial management of patients with operable colerectal cancer. In: Wagener DJ (ed) Chemotherapy preceding surgery or irradiation in cancer medicine. Liss, New York (in press).

Ries J, Ludwig H, Appel W (1968) Anticoagulants in the radiation treatment of carcinoma of the female genitalia. Med Welt 38: 2042-2047

Rohwedder JJ, Sagastume E (1977) Heparin and polychemotherapy for treatment of lung cancer. Cancer Treat Rep 61: 1399-1401

Schabel FM (1975) Concepts for systemic treatment of micrometastases. Cancer 35: 15-24

Schaeffer JR (1964) Interference in localization of I^{131} fibrinogen in rat tumors by anticoagulants. Am J Physiol 206: 573-579

Schultz RM, Papamatheakis JD, Chirigos MA (1977) Interferon: an inducer of macrophage activation by polyanions. Science 197: 674-676

Suemasu K (1970) Inhibitive effect of heparin and dextran sulfate on experimental pulmonary metastases. Gann 61: 125

Taylor I (1981) Studies on the treatment and prevention of colorectal liver metastases. Ann R Coll Surg Engl 63: 270-273

Thornes RD (1972) Fibrin and cancer. Br Med J 1: 110

Thornes RD (1974) Oral anticoagulant therapy of human cancer. J Med 5: 83-91

Waddell WR (19737) Chemotherapy for carcinoma of the pancreas. Surgery 74: 420

Welch JP, Donaldson GA (1974) Recent experiences in the management of cancer of the colon and rectum. Am J Surg 127: 258-266

Williams JRB, Maugham E (1972) Treatment of tumor metastases by defibrination. Br Med J 3: 174

Zacharski LR, Henderson WG, Rickles FR, Forman WB, Cornell CJ Jr, Forcier RJ, Harrower HW, Johnson RO (1979) Rationale and experimental design for the VA cooperative study of anticoagulation (warfarin) in the treatment of cancer. Cancer 44: 732-741

Preoperative Chemotherapy for Gastric Cancer: A Prospective Study with at Least 1 Year Follow-up

A. N. Papaioannou, J. A. Kozonis, A. P. Polychronis, J. Nomicos, G. A. Plataniotis, and J. K. Papageorgiou

Department of Surgery, Mount Vernon Hospital, 12 North Seventh Avenue, Mount Vernon, NY 10550, USA

Introduction

Despite its declining incidence gastric cancer (GC) continues to be an important cause of death in the Western world (Papaioannou 1981 b). As a rule, the disease presents itself late, not being amenable to possible cure by presently available means. In a recent report, for example, among 192 patients who were explored, 80 operations were considered to be "curative" and only 7 were "early" cases. The overall 5-year survival in this series was 5.6% (Scott et al. 1985). It is obvious that surgery alone is not sufficient to deal with this disease, irrespective of how radical it may be. Adjuvant chemotherapy in a variety of schemes and schedules tested prospectively has also been unsuccessful (Rake et al. 1976; Kingstone et al. 1978; Dent et al. 1979). On the basis of the above evidence, 5 years ago we suggested that the possible reasons for our failure to improve end results, even in relatively early cases of GC, may be the early micrometastatic dissemination of the disease, which may, in fact, become enhanced during gastrectomy. This was considered likely as a result of the immunosuppression due to surgical stress and anesthesia as well as the influence of other perioperative tumor-promoting events modifying the subsequent course of the disease. To minimize or prevent this occurrence, was suggested that GC must be conceptually accepted as a systemic disease and treated initially by systemic chemotherapy (Papaioannou 1981 b). Unfortunately, the idea has been unattractive to surgeons and the formation of a collaborative group to gather a sizeable group of patients has not become possible. We are, therefore, reporting here a small prospectively randomized series of GC patients from one surgical service alone, where the principle of preoperative chemotherapy (PrCh) was tested and all patients have been followed for at least 1 year.

Patients, Methods, and Results

Patients with adenocarcinoma of any part of the stomach were alternatingly allocated to receive one cycle before and five cycles of chemotherapy after gastrectomy (study group), or have all six cycles postoperatively (control group). The following agents were used:

Cycles I, III, V: 5-fluorouracil 650 mg/m^2, Adriamycin 30 mg/m^2, mitomycin C 10 mg/m^2
Cycles II, IV, VI: 5-fluorouracil 650 mg/m^2, Adriamycin 50 mg/m^2

Study patients received cycle I 3 weeks before operation and continued with cycle II as soon after gastrectomy as feasible (usually after 2 weeks). Patients found to have metastatic disease to the liver or elsewhere, except in lymph nodes, either during the preoperative workup or at exploration, were excluded. An attempt was initially made to assess endo-

Recent Results in Cancer Research. Vol 103

scopically the effect of PrCh. However, changes in the size or other visible characteristics of the tumor could not be appreciated and this effort was later abandoned as unproductive. Ten patients were allocated in each group after completion of their workup. The men-to-women ratio was equal in both groups. With regard to the clinical stage of the disease, based on the UICC classification, the study group was slightly weighted with more advanced cases in terms of gross extent of disease and of lymph node metastases. All patients had mechanical catharsis of the bowel either with the standard protocol of low-residue diet, cathartics, and enemas, or through whole-gut irrigation. All patients were given one oral preoperative dose of metronidazole by mouth the night before operation and were begun on chloramphenicol the morning of operation. Chloramphenicol was continued 1 g every 8 h for 3 consecutive days thereafter. Patients who were given preoperative chemotherapy underwent gastrectomy 2-3 weeks later. The extent and type of gastrectomy done was appropriate for each case, to achieve tumor-free margins of resection. Grossly involved or suspiciously enlarged lymph nodes were removed but formal lymph node dissections were not done. An effort was made to save rather than resect the spleen unless it was in the immediate vicinity or actually involved by tumor. The spleen was not removed, for example, in one patient in the control group with carcinoma of the gastroesophageal junction. In one patient of the study group with very extensive disease, to gain tumor-free margins, resection was carried out so far that duodenal closure was not possible and directed duodenal fistula had to be constructed with a Foley catheter. There were no wound dehiscences or wound infections in either group. Drains, as a rule, were not placed. The operative time was on average 22 min shorter in the study group and the mean blood loss (as measured by the total amount of blood replaced during and after operation) was less by 460 ml in the study group (Table 1). This accorded with the impression gained by the operating surgeons of easier dissections and less bloody operations after chemotherapy. Histological changes suggestive of cellular damage could not be identified with certainty. In one study patient, however, although the primary tumor appeared to be poorly differentiated, its metastases in the only regional node they were identified were well differentiated. Succulent sinusoids and reactive hyperplasia could be seen in uninvolved nodes of the same patient. This patient is now doing very well nearly 2 years after operation. The types of gastrectomy done, the survival and other data, in each group, are shown in Table 1. The small numbers prevent achievement of real statistical significance. The trend in favor of PrCh is evident, however, in the improved survival of patients receiving PrCh and particularly in the prolongation of disease-free survival in patients in whom disease recurred.

Discussion

The usual presentation of GC at late stages, the inability of the so-called "curative" radical surgery to control the disease in the majority of instances (Scott et al. 1985), and the frequently delayed recrudescence of the disease even in patients thought to be cured 3 years after gastrectomy, as it was documented in the study of Serlin et al. (1977), represent sufficient evidence to suggest that GC is a systemic diesease in most instances at the time of diagnosis. Since existing evidence strongly suggests enhancement of micrometastases, occurring perioperatively, it is possible that during gastrectomy existing micrometastases become entrenched and the establishment of new ones is facilitated in the favorable climate of immunosuppression. Hypercoagulability, and other tumor-enhancing factors prevail in the perioperative period (Papaioannou 1981 a).

Table 1. Results of preoperative chemotherapy in gastric cancer

Type of gastrectomy	Study (*n*, 10)		Control (*n*, 10)
	Pr=1; B1=4; B2=5		T=1; Pr=1; B1=3; B2=5
Mean operative time (min)	155		177
Mean blood loss (ml)	510		970
Deaths	5		5
Mean survival alive NED (months)	33.5		22.5
Mean survival NED to recurrence (months)	11.2	$P<0.1$	5.75

T, total; *B*, Billroth; *Pr*, proximal; *NED*, no evidence of disease

The many ways in which administration of chemotherapy is more advisable before rather than after resection of operable solid tumors have been recently discussed (Papaioannou 1981 a, 1984). The arguments in support of PrCh can be summarized as follows: tumors obeying Gompertzian kinetics have their highest chemosensitivity point at the time of their maximal growth rate, which is at the inflection point of the Gompertzian curve (Norton and Simon 1977). Likewise, a new theory (Goldie and Coldman 1979) based on the spontaneous development of chemoresistant clones expected to occur by random mutation during the natural history of any tumor places the greatest changes for chemotherapeutic success at the earliest possible moment chemotherapy may be administered.

An important practical advantage of PrCh is the in vivo assessment of chemosensitivity for tumors that can be directly or indirectly measured. Tumor response to chemotherapy is a highly complex phenomenon occurring in vivo (Watson 1981), only a small part of which can be evaluated in any in vitro chemosensitivity test. Clinically measurable tumor responses were predictive of subsequent recurrence following PrCh in patients with osteogenic sarcoma (Frei 1983), but only partially so in patients with stage III breast cancer (Papaioannou et al. 1983). However, if the tumor is initially resected, the opportunity to assess the in vivo chemosensitivity is lost and postoperative adjuvant chemotherapy is continued blindly for months or years until the recurrence becomes clinically evident. Furthermore, the possibility of reduction in patient survival exists, if appropriate therapy is not instituted at the earliest possible time, when such treatment is more likely to be successful (Schabel 1975) If operation precedes chemotherapy, the micrometastatic burden, possibly present to some extent in all solid tumors, is given an opportunity to increase in size particularly under the conditions of immunosuppression and the influence of other tumor-enhancing factors at work in the perioperative period. In addition, the smaller the neoplastic focus the greater the likelihood for the neoplastic cells to be better oxygenated, to divide more actively, and to accumulate fewer metabolites inhibiting the efficacy of chemotherapeutic agents. Effectiveness of chemotherapy is therefore more likely at this early stage (Papaioannou 1981 a).

Following the initial immunosuppressive phase induced by chemotherapeutic agents, immunity not only recovers, but in fact exceeds, its initial strength present before chemotherapy. This phenomenon, known as "immunological overshoot," can be exploited clinically as a means of nonspecific immunostimulation by timing the operative procedure during that phase. By using PrCh in that way, the immunosuppressive effects of trauma, anesthesia, etc., are, at least partly, counteracted. Furthermore, if cells in the primary tumor destined to form metastases enter the circulation during surgical manipulations with intact potential, they would be more likely to take foothold, particularly in the state of postoperative hypercoagulability and immunosuppression, both of which favor the establishment of new metastases. If, however, their potential is diminished or eliminated by PrCh, the possibility of new micrometastases developing as a result of surgical manipulations is reduced. Finally, after PrCh, operations are made easier and the saving of blood and operative time may be appreciable, because the size and vascularity of the primary tumors treated by PrCh are reduced and their resectability is improved (Papaioannou 1981 a).

Experimentally, the efficacy of PrCh has been shown since at least 25 years ago (Brock 1959) and has been demonstrated in a variety of experimental animal tumor systems (Karrer et al. 1967; Bogden et al. 1974; Schabel et al. 1974; Pendergrast and Futrell 1979; Osteen and Wilson 1980; Fisher et al. 1979; Van Putten 1985).

Clinically, there are two trials in breast cancer and one in gastric cancer supporting the efficacy of perioperative adjuvant chemotherapy. The first study is the earliest large-scale breast collaborative trial in the United States, testing thiotepa given during mastectomy and during the first two postoperative days. Ten years after the study was initiated premenopausal patients with four or more positive nodes given thiotepa were found to have a 20% survival advantage over untreated controls (Fisher et al. 1968). The second study is a Scandinavian cooperative trial using a 6-day course of cyclophosphamide starting on the day of mastectomy (Nissen-Meyer et al. 1981). Radiotherapy followed in all patients. In one institution, however, this chemotherapy course was delayed by 2-4 weeks to have radiotherapy completed first. Statistically, the cyclophosphamide-treated patients had a significantly better survival than controls, which was maintained for over 12 years, except in patients whose chemotherapy was delayed. Was this approximate 3-week delay in instituting chemotherapy responsible for the loss of chemotherapeutic effectiveness of the regimen? We believe this to be so and we have suggested that a likely explanation for this observation is that metastases become more vulnerable to chemotherapy immediately after the resection of the primary tumor, because their growth rate is accelerated usually for a short period only. This very interesting and largely unexplained phenomenon to our knowledge occurs in almost all experimental settings in which it has so far been studies. If the same kinetic change occurs in man, the immediate postoperative period may be the most sensitive phase in the natural history of operable tumors, as well as possibly the one that we may be most capable to intervene on effectively. (For review see Papaioannou et al. 1985.) PrCh was also given prospectively in 1805 Japanese GC patients in four different schedules. Patients with stage III GC and those with lymph node metastases who received bolus mitomycin C (MMC) the day of gastrectomy and the following day (total 30 mg) plus ftorafur for 3 months starting 1 month after operation had a survival advantage over those not receiving ftorafur (Inokuchi et al. 1984). They also had an even better survival over those who received the same schedule but with the MMC not in bolus form but in small doses every 2 weeks after operation for 4-5 weeks. The perioperative MMC bolus, compared with the low postoperative dose, is superior in almost each subset of patients given. Thus, the immediate postoperative period may well be a more advantageous phase to render chemotherapy effective than 2-4 weeks later, as it is routinely practiced today in most adjuvant chemotherapy programs treating solid tumors postoperatively. The loss of efficacy of chemotherapeutic regimen if given 3 weeks after mastectomy, as in the Scandinavian trial, or in low instead of high doses, immediately after gastrectomy as in the Japanese trial, strongly supports this notion.

The choice of chemotherapeutic regimen for carcinoma of the stomach in our trial was influenced by the efficacy of the FAM regimen (5-fluorouracil, Adriamycin, and mitomycin C) in patients with advanced gastric carcinoma.

In the present study, the limited numbers available prevent any conclusions, but the trends in favor of PrCh are obvious as shown in Table 1. The mean survival without evidence of disease is better in the study group and likewise the disease-free interval of those who received PrCh but ultimately developed recurrence is double that of their counterparts in the control group. In addition, the administration of PrCh appears to be advantageous from an operative point of view. Operations, in fact, became easier and less bloody after PrCh and, therefore, their duration was decreased. Infections, wound problems, or other major complications were not encountered. PrCh may, therefore, be considered safe. Insofar as effectiveness is concerned, it is possible that more than one cycle, possibly two, or even three cycles of chemotherapy are needed before operation to make a better impact on the systemic component of the disease. This, however, remains to be studied. In our view, it is rather unlikely that PrCh may, in fact, have a very marked impact on the ultimate prospects of any solid tumor that usually presents itself late. As pointed out by Goldie and Coldman (1979), the chances of chemoresistant clones developing in any tumor, irrespective of its growth rate, increase very rapidly over a very short span of the natural history of growth of that tumor. Chemoresistant clones may, therefore, well exist at the time of diagnosis in the majority of instances, thus negating any efforts of preoperative and postoperative chemotherapy alike.

Not to conclude in that pessimistic tone despite the above possibility, we believe that PrCh represents a very worthwhile concept that may push the frontiers back, particularly in tumors with a longer range of survival. It may well be that with an increased number of PrCh cycles a greater tumor shrinkage will occur, as we have shown with two preoperative cycles in stage III breast cancer (Papaioannou et al. 1983, 1985), hopefully reflecting a more effective impact on the all important micrometastases. If this occurs, the extent of operations as well as their untoward effects on host resistance mechanisms may be minimized so that the latter may effect "cure" by killing remaining chemoresistant clones. The major challenge in this area is probably the difficulty in modifying physician attitudes sufficiently to make them accept change and contribute their patients to well-organized cooperative efforts to answer the important questions raised in this conference.

Acknowledgment. I am indebted to Dr. James Spencer, Head of the Department of Pathology at Mount Vernon Hospital, for help in the interpretation of histological material.

References

Bogden AF, Esher HJ, Taylor DJ, Gray JH (1974) Comparative study on the effect of surgery, chemotherapy and immunotherapy alone and in combination on metastases of the 13762 mammary adenocarcinoma. Cancer Res 34: 1627-1630

Brock H (1959) Neue experimentelle Ergebnisse mit *N*-lostphosphamidestern. Strahlentherapie 41: 347-353

Dent DM, Werner ID, Novis B, Cheverton P, Brize P (1979) Prospecitve randomized trial of combined oncological therapy for gastric carcinoma. Cancer 44: 385

Fisher B, Ravdin RG, Ausman RK, Slack NH, Moore GE, Noer RJ, Cooperating Investigators (1968) Surgical adjuvant chemotherapy in cancer of the breast: results of a decade of cooperative investigations. Ann Surg 168: 337-343

Fisher R, Gerhardt M, Saffer E (1979) Effect of treatment prior to primary tumor removal on the growth of distal tumor. Cancer 43: 451-459

Frei E III (1983) Clinical cancer research: an embattled species. Cancer 50: 1979-1982

Goldie JH, Coldman AJ (1979) A mathematical model for relating the drug sensitivity of tumors to their spontaneous mutation rate. Cancer treat Rep 63: 1727-1730

Inokuchi K, Hattori T, Taguchi T, Abe O, Ogawa N (1984) Postoperative adjuvant chemotherapy for gastric carcinoma. Analysis of data of 1805 patients followed for 5 years. Cancer 53: 2393-2397

Karrer K, Humphreys SR, Goldin A (1967) An experimental model for studying factors which influence metastases of malignant tumors. Int J Cancer 2: 213-218

Kingstone RD, Ellis DJ, Brooke VS, Waterhouse JAH, Hwist MD, Smith JA (1978) The West Midlands gastric carcinoma chemotherapy trial: planning and results. Clin Oncol 4: 55-59

Nissen-Meyer R, Kjelgren K, Melmoik B, et al (1981) Surgical adjuvant chemotherapy with one single 6-day cyclophosphamide course: 12-year follow-up. Advances in medical oncology research and education, vol 12. Pergamon, Oxford, pp 1177-1179

Norton L, Simon R (1977) Tumor size, sensitivity of therapy and design of treatment schedules. Cancer Treat Rep 61: 1307-1317

Osteen RT, Wilson RE (1980) The timings of surgery and chemotherapy in an animal tumor model. 33rd Annual meeting of the Society of Surgical Oncology, San Francisco, May 14, 1980

Papaioannou AN (1981 a) Perspectives in cancer research: preoperative chemotherapy for operable solid tumors. Eur J Cancer 17: 963-969

Papaioannou AN (1981 b) Why do we fail in gastric cancer: what can we do about it? In: Friedman M, Ogawa M, Kisner D (eds) Diagnosis and treatment of upper gastrointestinal tumors. International Congress Series 542. Excerpta Medica, Amsterdam, pp 237-252

Papaioannou AN (1984) Systemic therapy as the initial step in the management of operable breast cancer. Surg Clin North Am 64: 1181-1191

Papaioannou AN, Kozonis J, Polychronis A, Papagerogiou G, Lissaios B, Kondylis D, Vasilaros S, Papadiamantis J, Tsiliakos S, Razis D, Throuvalas N, Papavassilious K, Sakelaris J, Tsarouhas CH, Collaborating Investigators of the Hellenic Breast Cooperative Group (HBCG) (1983) Shrinkage of stage III, primary breast cancer (BC) to preoperative (preop) systemic therapy (Rx). Presented at the 3rd EORTC Cancer Working Conference, April 28, 1983, Amsterdam. Abstract IX

Papaioannou AN, Kozonis J, Polychronis A, other Collaborating Investigators of the Hellenic Breast Cooperative Group (1985) Preoperative chemotherapy. Advantages and clinical application in stage III breast cancer. In: Senn HJ, Metzger U (eds) Adjuvent chemotherapy of breast cancer. Springer, Berlin Heidelber New York (Recent results in cancer research, vol 96)

Pendergrast WJ Jr, Futrell JW (1979) Biologic determination of tumor growth in healing wounds. Ann Surg 189: 181-188

Rake MO, Mallison CN, Cocking BJ, Cynaski RT, Fox C, Jackson A, Diffey B (1976) Assessment of the value of cytotoxic therapy in the treatment of carcinoma of the stomach. Gut 17: 832

Schabel FM (1975) Concepts for systemic treatment of micrometastases. Cancer 35: 15-25

Schabel FM Jr, Griswold DP Jr, Corbett TH, Laster WR Jr, Dyker DJ, Rose WC (1974) Recent studies with adjuvant chemotherapy or immunotherapy of metastatic solid tumors of mice. In: Jones SE, Salmon SE (eds) Adjuvant therapy of cancer II. Grune and Stratton, New York, pp 476-488

Scott HW Jr, Adkins RB Jr, Sawyer JL (1985) Results of an aggressive surgical approach to gastric carcinoma during a twenty-three year period. Surgery 97: 55-59

Serlin D, Dahn RJ, Higgins GA Jr, Harrower HW, Mandeloff GL (1977) Factors related to survival following resection for gastric carcinoma. Cancer 40: 1318-1331

Van Putten LM (to be published) Optimal timing of adjuvant chemotherapy for mouse tumors. In: Wagener DJ (ed) Chemotherapy preceding surgery or irradiation in cancer medicine. Liss, New York

Watson JV (1981) What does "response" in cancer chemotherapy really mean? Br Med J II: 34-37

Neoadjuvant Chemotherapy for Osteogenic Sarcoma: A Model for the Treatment of Other Highly Malignant Neoplasms

G. Rosen

Comprehensive Cancer Center Inc., Beverly Hills, Los Angeles, CA, USA

Introduction

The term "neoadjuvant chemotherapy" was first described by Frei in his Karnofsky lecture, where it was used to describe the use and benefits of preoperative chemotherapy for the treatment of malignant tumors (Frei 1982). An early example of the use of neoadjuvant or preoperative chemotherapy was in the development of effective treatment for osteogenic sarcoma, the most common malignant bone tumor seen in the adolescent and young adult population (Rosen et al. 1982). The advantages of neoadjuvant chemotherapy on theoretical grounds would appear to be the early elimination of metastatic microfoci of disease that exist in the majority of patients harboring fully malignant (ostensibly only) primary malignant tumors. Early aggressive therapy theoretically would not only destroy metastatic microfoci of disease that exists systemically, but by the use of aggressive chemotherapy that can cause regression of the primary tumor, presumably the emergence of resistant tumor cells would be prevented.

The early use of full doses of aggressive chemotherapy to rid the body of systemic micrometastases and prevent the emergence of resistant cell lines is, however, only one advantage of neoadjuvant chemotherapy. That one advantage would presumably be gained by the patient who had a complete response of his or her primary tumor to preoperative chemotherapy. Even in the best of circumstances, most primary tumors treated with preoperative chemotherapy would at best be expected to have only a 50% complete response rate to preoperative chemotherapy. How then does preoperative or neoadjuvant chemotherapy benefit the patient who does not have a complete response? In order to be valuable for all patients, neoadjuvant or preoperative chemotherapy has to address the latter point as well.

In the model developed for the treatment of osteogenic sarcoma, another advantage of neoadjuvant chemotherapy is application of the response of the primary tumor to determine postoperative or classic "adjuvant" chemotherapy. In this model, patients not having a complete response to preoperative chemotherapy with high-dose methotrexate and leucovorin rescue and the combination of bleomycin, cyclophosphamide, and dactinomycin (BCD) were given alternative chemotherapy with cisplatin in combination with Adriamycin. The early application of this newly proven effective phase II combination of drugs for adjuvant chemotherapy in patients that did not have a complete response of their primary tumor to the standard high-dose methotrexate and BCD chemotherapy greatly increased the disease-free survival in that group of patients not responding well to preoperative chemotherapy.

Thus, the ability to choose alternative best second-line or newly found effective chemotherapy for a disease following the demonstrated failure of standard chemotherapy for

Recent Results in Cancer Research. Vol 103

that disease to effect a complete response in the primary tumor has led to further advances in the treatment of that disease. This is a second theoretical and practical advantage of the use of preoperative or neoadjuvant chemotherapy.

Methods

Effective chemotherapy for metastatic osteogenic sarcoma evolved in the early 1970s. Although Adriamycin given at the dose of 90 mg/m^2 was felt to be effective in the treatment of osteogenic sarcoma (Cortes et al. 1975), in this author's experience the most effective treatment for metastatic osteogenic sarcoma was high-dose methotrexate with leucovorin rescue originally described by Jaffe et al. (1978). An early pilot adjuvant chemotherapy protocol (T-4) utilized high-dose methotrexate at the dose of 200 mg/m^2 for all patients, and Adriamycin and cyclophosphamide (Rosen et al. 1976). It was noted, however, in the early use of preoperative chemotherapy with this protocol that the majority of the younger patients did not respond to preoperative chemotherapy with high-dose methotrexate at that dose. In September 1976 a preoperative chemotherapy protocol (T-7) was initiated utilizing high-dose methotrexate at the dose of 8 g/m^2 for fully grown adolescents and adults and 12 g/m^2 for younger children. This latter 12 g/m^2 dose seemed to cause regression of metastatic disease as well as primary tumors in the younger children (Rosen et al. 1979). In addition, the combination of bleomycin (15 mg/m^2 per day for 2 days), cyclophosphamide (600 mg/m^2 per day for 2 days), and dactinomycin (0.6 mg/m^2 per day for 2 days) was also incorporated into the protocol, since it had been shown to be effective in the treatment of metastatic osteogenic sarcoma as well (Mosende et al. 1977). The T-7 protocol also incorporated the use of Adriamycin at the dose of 30 mg/m^2 per day for 3 days. This protocol called for preoperative chemotherapy in all patients and is depicted in

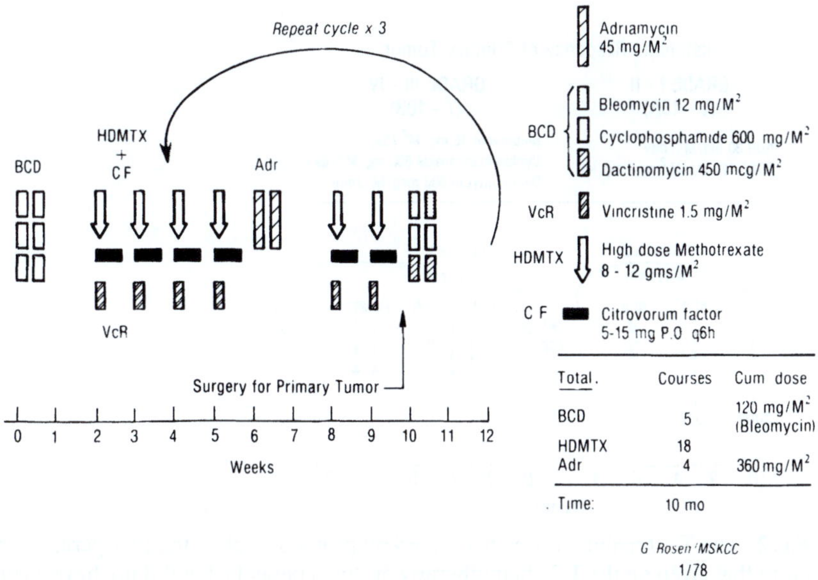

Fig. 1. The T-7 chemotherapy protocol started in 1976. The dose of dactinomycin was subsequently raised to 0.6 mg/m^2 per day for 2 days. Of the 37 patients treated on this protocol, 26 had a complete response of their primary tumor to preoperative chemotherapy

Table 1. Preoperative chemotherapy for primary osteogenic sarcoma

Histological response of primary tumor to chemotherapy
I. No discernible effect
II. Partial effect: > 50% of specimen No tumor cells (*areas* of tumor cells detected)
III. Good effect: > 90% of specimen No tumor cells (small *foci* of tumor cells detected)
IV. Complete effect: 100% of specimen No tumor cells detected

Fig. 1. The dose of dactinomycin (450 mg/m^2) described in the figure was subsequently changed to 600 mg or 0.6 mg/m^2 per day for 2 days.

After preoperative chemotherapy, patients had surgery (either amputation or resection). Following surgery, the entire specimen was sectioned and examined for the histological effect of preoperative chemotherapy on the primary tumor. Patients having a complete response to preoperative chemotherapy were designated as those who had either no viable tumor cells detected in the entire specimen (grade IV) or those patients that had greater than 90% of the specimen showing absolutely no tumor cells, but small foci or tumor cells detected in a few microscopic areas of the tumor (grade III). The histological grading of the response of the primary tumor to preoperative chemotherapy is shown in Table 1.

As the T-7 chemotherapy protocol progressed, it was noted that all patients that had a grade III or grade IV effect of preoperative chemotherapy on the primary tumor were disease-free survivors. Relapses took place in patients having either no effect of preoperative chemotherapy on the primary tumor or a good partial effect of preoperative chemotherapy on the primary tumor. In the latter instance, microscopic areas of confluent tumor cells were found as residue in the primary tumor even though it otherwise responded well

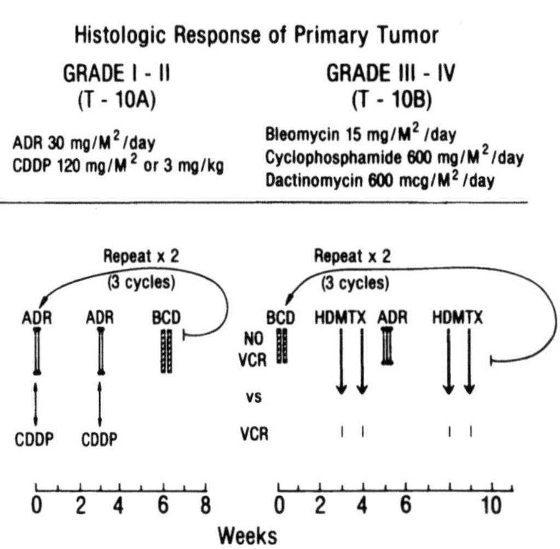

Fig. 2. The T-10 maintenance chemotherapy protocol. Following preoperative chemotherapy similar to that given on the T-7 chemotherapy protocol patients that did not have a complete response of the primary tumor to preoperative chemotherapy received regimen T-10A or basically Adriamycin combined with displatin. Patients responding completely to preoperative chemotherapy with high-dose methotrexate, BCD, and Adriamycin continued on the same regimen (T-10B) postoperatively

to preoperative chemotherapy with high-dose methotrexate. In retrospect, these residual areas of tumor probably represented the emergence of resistant tumor cells, since even those patients having an almost 90% or better response to the primary tumor to preoperative chemotherapy were at risk of relapse if they had confluent areas of tumor cells occupying the majority of any of the multiple sections following histological analysis of the resected tumor.

In mid-1978, it becamed apparent that the combination of Adriamycin and cisplatin was effective in the treatment of metastatic osteogenic sarcoma (Ettinger et al. 1981; Rosen et al. 1980). Thus at that time, it was decided to add Adriamycin to the dose of 60 mg/m^2 given over 2 days combined with cisplatin at the dose of 120 mg/m^2 given with a mannitol diuresis in the postoperative treatment of only patients who did not have complete response of their tumor to preoperative chemotherapy with high-dose methotrexate, Adriamycin, and BCD following histological analysis of the resected specimen. This then evolved into the T-10 chemotherapy protocol which allowed for the selection of alternative postoperative adjuvant chemotherapy with Adriamycin and cisplatin for those patients who did not respond completely to preoperative chemotherapy (Rosen et al. 1982). On the other hand, the complete responders to preoperative chemotherapy continued on the same chemotherapy as was given preoperatively; namely, BCD, high-dose methotrexate, and Adriamycin (Fig. 2).

In November 1981, in an attempt to limit the toxicity and cost of treatment, the question was posed "Do we need to continue prolonged postoperative chemotherapy in patients who have a complete response of their primary tumor to preoperative chemotherapy?" this brought about the proposal of a new protocol in which patients that had a complete response of the primary tumor to preoperative chemotherapy with high-dose methotrexate and BCD would be randomized either to continue the same chemotherapy postopera-

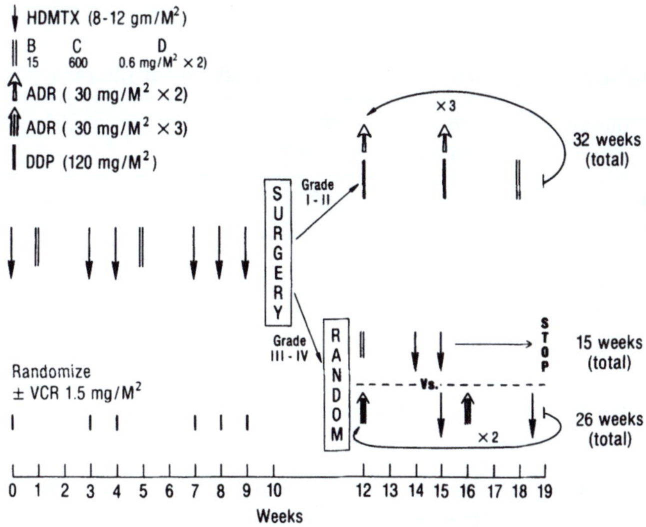

Fig. 3. The proposed T-12 chemotherapy protocol attempted to stop patients after only 15 weeks of chemotherapy with BCD and high-dose methotrexate if they had a complete response of the primary tumor to that same chemotherapy given preoperatively. The randomization was not done since this protocol was run as a pilot study and should now be proposed as a randomized study for cooperative groups to determine the efficacy of the early discontinuation of chemotherapy in good responding patients

tively or stop therapy early at 15 weeks after only one more BCD and two high-dose methotrexate treatments given post-operatively. This was designated as the T-12 chemotherapy protocol (Fig. 3). However, since this study was to be done at a single institution, it was determined that it would take too long to perform the randomized study, and it was decided to run the T-12 protocol offering the short arm of chemotherapy (stopping at 15 weeks) to patients who had a complete response of their primary tumor to preoperative chemotherapy with BCD and high-dose methotrexate. Therefore, randomization was not done and the T-12 chemotherapy protocol was run as a pilot in 51 patients. Those having a complete response of preoperative chemotherapy received only one BCD treatment and two high-dose methotrexate treatments postoperatively. The advantage of this approach to the treatment of osteogenic sarcoma would be that it enabled us to shorten the course of post-operative or adjuvant chemotherapy in patients who have a complete response to preoperative chemotherapy and avoid the use of the potentially toxic agents Adriamycin and cisplatin.

The exact details of each of the chemotherapy protocols as well as the intricate details of the administration of high-dose methotrexate with leucovorin rescue have been previously reported in detail (Nirenberg et al. 1977, Rosen et al. 1976, 1979, 1982; Rosen 1985).

Results

From September 1976 through November 1983, 175 patients were given preoperative chemotherapy on T-7, T-10, and T-12 protocol. The overall results are shown in Table 2. Of the 175 patients, 133 remain alive and continuously free of disease (76%); 140 patients are currently alive and free of disease (7 patients developing solitary metastasis have been salvaged with further surgery and chemotherapy) for an overall disease-free survival of 80% at a median time of 52 months. During the past decade limb salvage surgery has be-

Table 2. Preoperative chemotherapy for osteogenic sarcoma

Protocol	No. of patients	No. with CDFS	%	No. ANED	%	Median time (months)
T-7	37	28	76	30	81	89
T-10	87	67	77	71	82	58
T-12	51	38	75	39	76	25
Total	175	133	76	140	80	52

CDFS, continuous disease-free survival; *ANED*, alive with no evidence of disease

Table 3. Preoperative chemotherapy for osteogenic sarcoma excluding 12 patients with documented local recurrences

Protocol	No. of patients	No. with CDFS	%	No. ANED	%
T-7	33	28	85	30	91
T-10	85	67	79	71	84
T-12	45	38	84	38	84
Total	163	133	82	139	85

CDFS, continuous disease-free survival; *ANED*, alive with no evidence of disease

come more popular. One of the risks of limb salvage surgery is, of course, local recurrence, and careful criteria for the selection of patients for such surgery must be exercised in patients with osteogenic sarcoma. In our 175 patients given preoperative chemotherapy, 120 of the patients underwent limb salvage surgery during the study period. During that period there were 12 local recurrences (10%). In order to examine the efficacy of neoadjuvant chemotherapy it would be useful to examine the results of treatment excluding the 12 patients that had documented local recurrences (Table 3). In that group of 163 patients, 133, or 82%, are continuously alive and free of disease at a median time of over 4 years, and 85% of the patients are currently surviving free of disease.

In the data reported in Tables 2 and 3, there is apparently no difference between the T-7, T-10, and T-12 protocol results. However, it should be noted that the number of patients treated on T-7 is small (37) and to our good fortune 26 of those 37 patients (70%) had complete responses of their primary tumor to preoperative chemotherapy. Whereas in the larger group of 138 patients on the T-10 and T-12 protocol only 49% of the patients had complete responses of their primary tumor to preoperative chemotherapy. Clearly the addition of cisplatin and Adriamycin for the patients not having a complete response to high-dose methotrexate preoperative chemotherapy has made a difference in survival in the poor-prognosis subset of patients, although it does not appear to be reflected in the overall results of the three treatment protocols.

The apparent equality in the overall disease-free survival of patients treated on the pilot T-12 chemotherapy protocol as compared with the T-10 chemotherapy protocol indicates that the lack of difference in outcome may allow us to stop chemotherapy early in those patients achieving a complete response to preoperative chemotherapy with high-dose methotrexate and BCD chemotherapy.

Discussion

Although there has been some recent controversy about the utility of chemotherapy in the treatment of osteogenic sarcoma (Carter 1984, Edmonson et al. 1984), that controversy has recently been put to rest by a randomized study conducted by the Pediatric Oncology Group in the United States, where there was a highly significant difference in survival between those patients receiving postoperative adjuvant chemotherapy and those receiving no chemotherapy. The results were highly significant, and the study had to be stopped because the survival of patients not receiving adjuvant chemotherapy was less than 10% (Link 1984).

Although this author had reported disease-free survival rates in excess of 80% with modern third-generation chemotherapy utilizing the proper dose of high-dose methotrexate (12 g/m^2 in younger children and 8 g/m^2 in adults) (Rosen et al. 1982), other groups not using this regimen had reported disease-free survival rates in the 50%–60% range (Cortes et al. 1979; Pratt et al. 1977). However, studies utilizing the drug doses originally recommended in the T-7 and T-10 chemotherapy protocols confirmed our early results; namely, the German-Austrian cooperative osteogenic sarcoma study (COSS-80) reported by Winkler et al. confirmed the fact that preoperative chemotherapy was of value in patients treated with osteogenic sarcoma, and that increasing the dose of methotrexate to 12 g/m^2 for younger children produced superior results over that obtained in their earlier first-generation study (COSS-77) (Winkler et al. 1984). In a recent report from Paris, Kalifa et al. was able almost exactly to duplicate the results obtained with the T-10 chemotherapy protocol when that protocol was used as originally described in 1982. In that report,

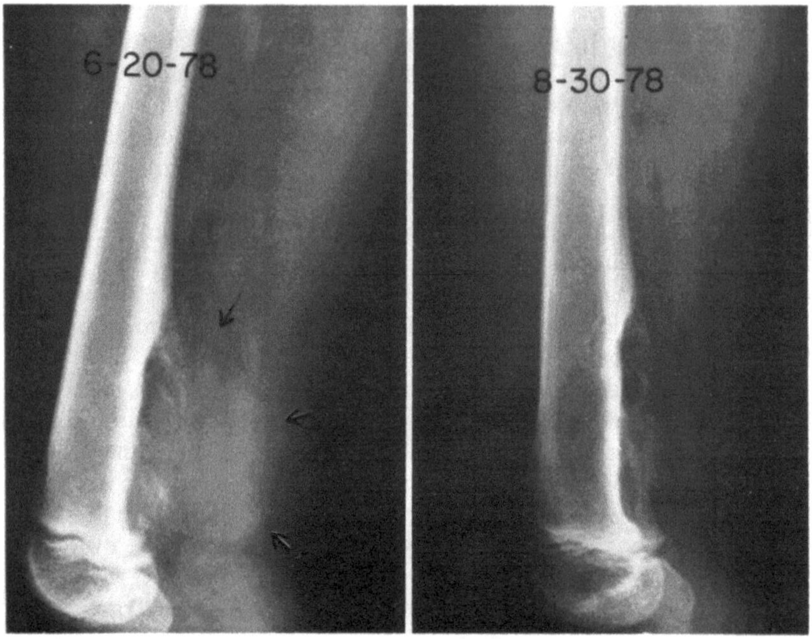

Fig. 4. Ostoegenic sarcoma of the distal femur with a large soft tissue mass prior to, and following, preoperative chemotherapy on the T-10 chemotherapy protocol. After 2 months of chemotherapy there was complete dissolution of the soft tissue mass and return of the normal fascial fat planes to their normal state. This facilitated resection surgery. In addition, this patient showed a complete response to preoperative chemotherapy following histological examination of the resected specimen. The patient is currently alive and continuously free of recurrent disease at 80 months from the start of treatment

Kalifa noted that 32 of 36 patients (89%) had a continuous disease-free survival at a median time of 20 months (Kalifa et al. 1985). In particular, the later study not only utilized the T-10 chemotherapy protocol as it was originally published, but the technique of giving high-dose methotrexate was also utilized as had been published previously (Rosen and Nirenberg 1982). Of note in other protocols using high-dose methotrexate, excessive intravenous fluid hydration is used, which was not used in the T-10 or T-12 protocol as originally described (Link 1984).

Preoperative chemotherapy should not be given by merely following a recipe. It is extremely important to follow the patient meticulously. It is not acceptable to have the patient put on a chemotherapy regimen and have the primary tumor progress while the patient is receiving apparently ineffective chemotherapy. While most primary tumors regress while undergoing preoperative chemotherapy (Fig. 4), occasionally the patient with osteogenic sarcoma who is not sensitive at all to high-dose methotrexate may witness some disease progression. It is important to document that treatment failure in order to take further steps either to expedite surgery or perhaps to take the patient off the treatment protocol and substitute best second-line therapy prior to surgery. Very useful in following patients on preoperative chemotherapy is the use of the gallium scan to evaluate tumor activity (Yeh et al. 1984). Future studies showing great promise will be the use of positron-emitting radionuclides. These substances have the advantage of a very low radiation dose to the patient and the ability to detect very early on changes in the metabolic rate of tu-

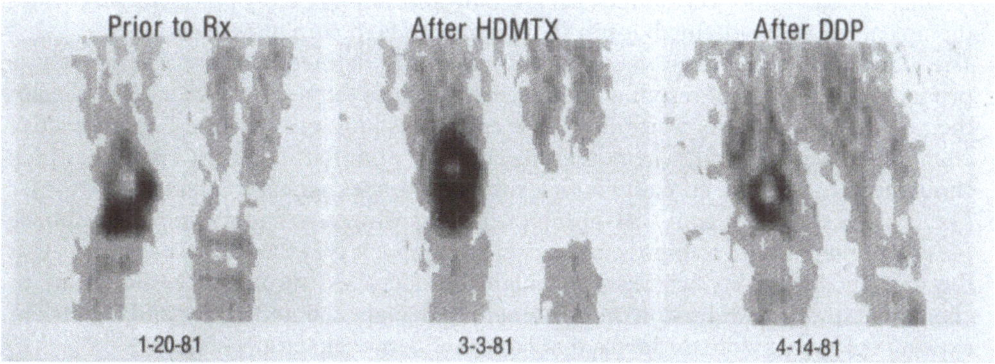

Fig. 5. Serial nitrogen-13 glutamate positron emission tomography images of a patient with osteogenic sarcoma of the distal femur. Although there was no clinical change in this patient, repeat imaging after four high-dose methotrexate treatments indicated that there was increased tumor metabolic activity in the distal femur lesion. At that point, the patient was switched to cisplatin in combination with Adriamycin and had regression of tumor. This allowed for the successful use of limb salvage surgery in this patient. The patient is still alive and free from recurrent disease at this time. This demonstrates the need for careful monitoring of patients while on preoperative chemotherapy. Use of sensitive detection devices such as positron emission imaging might allow us to titrate every patient to a complete response of the primary tumor while on preoperative chemotherapy. The response of the primary tumor will hopefully correlate with the patient's ultimate survival. Had this patient not been followed very closely, it is probable that a favorable outcome of treatment would not have been achieved

mors, which correlates with their response to chemotherapy (Reiman et al. 1982). In past years this has been an experimental technique confined to institutions that had the availability of cyclotrons to produce the positron-emitting radionuclides and a positron emission tomography apparatus. However, this type of technology will soon be made commercially available and should be an aid in administering preoperative chemotherapy at major institutions that acquire that technology. An example is demonstrated in Fig. 5, which demonstrates serial nitrogen-13 glutamate images of a primary osteogenic sarcoma. While undergoing preoperative chemotherapy, although clinically undetectable, N-13 scans indicated that the tumor appeared to be getting worse. In this particular patient (who wanted to have limb salvage surgery performed) preoperative chemotherapy was then switched to cisplatin, which then provided an immediate response, leading to the ability to perform limb salvage surgery. Thus newer imaging techniques, and perhaps the ability to utilize tumor markers that will be made available with new technology in monoclonal antibodies, will provide an even safer basis for the use of preoperative chemotherapy in the majority of patients with malignant neoplasms.

Thus in the past decade neoadjuvant, or preoperative, chemotherapy has made possible:

1. Definition of drugs and drug combinations that are active in the treatment of a particular disease.
2. Definition of the dose and timing of administration of those agents that cause optimal regression in the primary tumor and thus are optimal dose schedules to be used in adjuvant chemotherapy after primary tumor surgery.
3. The early eradication of microscopic foci of metastatic disease and the prevention of re-

sistant clones of tumor cells can be achieved by utilization of early preoperative chemotherapy at the above-defined doses, thus leading to high cure rates.
4. The identification of a high-risk group of patients as defined by those patients whose primary tumor does not respond completely to what is felt to be best standard chemotherapy for that disease. This allows the early substitution of second-line alternative chemotherapy or adjuvant chemotherapy early on, prior to the patient's relapse, which should lead to a higher cure rate in that subset of poor-prognosis patients.
5. The identification of a good-risk group of patients who have had a complete response of their primary tumor to preoperative chemotherapy. It is in this group of patients that the cost and morbidity of treatment might be decreased through the shortening of chemotherapy, the elimination of maintenance adjuvant chemotherapy, and the lack of exposure to more cytotoxic agents that have long-term deleterious effects.

The above criteria define the utility of and the raison d'être of "neoadjuvant" chemotherapy. This author believes that if neoadjuvant chemotherapy is able to deliver these theoretical concepts to the patient in his or her treatment, it will provide for advances in all areas of the treatment of malignant diseases within the next few years. It will also greatly accelerate the development of new and effective drug regimens for the treatment of cancer. Patients receiving neoadjuvant chemotherapy are certainly at no greater risk for not having immediate surgery, and indeed the use of preoperative chemotherapy has benefited the majority of patients receiving it.

References

Carter SK (1984) Adjuvant chemotherapy in osteogenic sarcoma: The triumph that isn't? J Clin Oncol 2 (3): 147-148

Cortes EP, Holland JF, Wang JJ, Glidewell O (1975) Adriamycin (NSC-123127), in 87 patients with osteogenic sarcoma. Cancer Chemother Rep 6: 305-313

Cortes EP, Necheles TF, Holland JF, et al (1979) Adriamycin (ADR) alone vs ADR and high-dose methotrexate-citrovorum factor rescue (HDM-CFR) ad adjuvant to operable primary osteosarcoma. A randomized study by Cancer and Leukemia Group B (CALGB). Proc Am Assoc Cancer Res 20: 412

Edmonson JH, Green SJ, Ivins JC, et al (1984) A controlled pilot study of high-dose methotrexate as postsurgical adjuvant treatment for primary osteosarcoma. J Clin Oncol 2 (3): 152-156

Ettinger LJ, Douglass HO, Highby DJ, et al. (1981) Adjuvant adriamycin (Adr) and cis-diamminedichloroplatinum (cis-platinum) in primary costesarcoma. Cancer 47: 248-254

Frei E (1982) Clinical cancer research: an embattled species. Cancer 50: 1979-1992

Jaffe N, Frei E, Watts H, et al (1978) High-dose methotrexate in osteogenic sarcoma. A 5-year experience. Cancer Treat Rep 62: 259-264

Kalifa C, Dubousset J, Contesso G, Vandel D, Lumbroso J, Lemerle J (1985) Osteosarcoma: an attempt to reproduce T-10 protocol in a single institution. Proc Am Soc Clin Onc 4: 236 (Abstr 919)

Link MP (1984) The role of adjuvant chemotherapy in the treatment of osteosarcoma of the extremity: preliminary results of the multi-institutional osteosarcoma study. Proceedings of National Institutes of Health Consensus Development Conference on Limb-sparing treatment: adult soft-tissue and osteogenic sarcomas. December 3-5, 1984, pp 74-78

Mosende C, Guittierez M, Caparros B, Rosen G (1977) Combination chemotherapy with bleomycin, cyclophosphamide and dactinomycin for the treatment of osteogenic sarcoma. Cancer 40: 2779-2786

Nirenberg A, Mosende C, Mehta BM, Gisolfi AL, Rosen G (1977) High dose methotrexate with citrovorum factor rescue: predictive value of serum methotrexate concentrations and corrective measures to avert toxicity. Cancer Treat Rep 61: 779-783

Pratt CB, Shanks EC, Hustu HO, et al (1977) Adjuvant multiple drug chemotherapy for esteogenic sarcoma of the extremity. Cancer 39: 51-57

Reiman RE, Rosen G, Gelbard AS, Benua, RS, Laughlin JS (1982) Imaging of primary Ewing sarcoma with 13N-l-glutamate. Radiology 42, (2): 495-500

Rosen G (1985) Chemotherapy for osteogenic sarcoma. In: Brian MC, Carbone PP (eds) Current therapy in hematology-oncology. Mosby, St. Louis, pp 217-224

Rosen G, Nirenberg A (1982) Chemotherapy for osteogenic sarcoma: an investigative method, not a recipe. Cancer Treat Rep 55: 1687-1697

Rosen G, Murphy ML, Huvos AG, et al (1976) Chemotherapy, en bloc resection and prosthetic bone replacement in the treatment of osteogenic sarcoma. Cancer 37: 1-11

Rosen G, Marcove RC, Caparros B, et al (1979) Primary osteogenic sarcoma. The rationale for preoperative chemotherapy and delayed surgery. Cancer 43: 2163-2177

Rosen G, Nirenberg A, Caparros B, et al (1980) Cis-platinum in metastatic osteogenic sarcoma. In: Prestayko AW, Crooke ST, Carter SK (eds) Cisplatin: current status and new developments. Academic, New York pp 465-475

Rosen G, Caparros B, Huvos AG, Kosloff C, Nirenberg A, Cacavio A, Marcova RC, Lane JM, Mehta B, Urban C (1982) Preoperative chemotherapy for osteogenic sarcoma: selection of postoperative adjuvant chemotherapy based on the response of the primary tumor to preoperative chemotherapy. Cancer 49: 1221-1230

Yeh SD, Rosen G, Caparros B, Benua RS (1984) Semiquantitative gallium scintigraphy in patients with osteogenic sarcoma. Clin Nucl Med 9: 175-183

Winkler K, Beron G, Kotz R, et al. (1984) Neoadjuvant chemotherapy for osteogenic sarcoma: results of a cooperative German/Austrian Study. J Clin Oncol 2 (6): 617-623

Summary of Preoperative (Neoadjuvant) Chemotherapy

J. M. Goldie, P. Band, and J. Ragaz

Cancer Control Agency of British Columbia, 600 West 10th Avenue, Vancouver, B. C. V5Z 4E6, Canada

The editors would like to express their appreciation to all of those who participated in this conference on neoadjuvant chemotherapy. It seems fair to summarize the general thrust of the papers presented by indicating that there do appear to be a number of sound theoretical reasons and preliminary clinical observations why preoperative chemotherapy would be beneficial. However, it must be conceded that definitive prospectively controlled studies for rigorous testing of the hypothesis have yet to be concluded, and hence that the final verdict on the utility of neoadjuvant chemotherapy must remain open.

There seems to be no arguing with the basic biological fact that small tumor burdens are much more likely to be curable by chemotherapy than are largeones. Surgical removal of a primary tumor leaves behind a relatively small residual population of microscopic metastatic disease. In experimental systems this maneuver can readily be shown to convert an incurable system into a curable one. This also appears to be true for a number of human malignancies. Therefore, the general utility of adjuvant chemotherapy in a number of disorders would seem to be established. The specific question being addressed during this meeting was whether advancing the timing of the adjuvant intervention to the earliest time feasible would result in measurable improvement in survival as compared to conventionally timed adjuvant chemotherapy.

There are at least three processes that have been discussed during the meeting that might be thought to be favorably influenced by early chemotherapy. Firstly, there is the question of drug resistance. In theoretical models as well as certain experimental systems, treatment delay by even a few tumor volume doubling times can have a significant impact on the probability of cure. This is related to the fact that the likelihood of appearance of the first resistance cell goes from a state of low to high probability over a relatively short interval in the tumor's growth history.

The next factor that may be involved is the overall growth kinetics of the micrometastatic disease. If the tumor during this time is growing more rapidly with a higher growth fraction, then its susceptibility to certain types of chemotherapeutic agents will be increased. For kinetic reasons the micrometastatic disease should be more susceptible to cure.

Lastly, another phenomenon which has been described in experimental systems is an enhanced growth rate seen in residual metastatic disease following removal of the primary tumor. The mechanism of this enhanced growth rate is uncertain, but in the absence of therapeutic intervention it might be reasonably inferred to be potentially deleterious to the host. Appropriately timed chemotherapy may abrogate this effect and in doing so neutralize a potentially adverse result of primary tumor extirpation. This phenomenon is seen in some experimental systems but not in others, and it is not clear at this time whether it has a counterpart in clinical malignancy. If it does, then it also raises the question of the appro-

Recent Results in Cancer Research. Vol 103

priate timing for the adjuvant chemotherapy - immediately prior to surgery or immediately after?

In addition to these theoretical benefits, two other potentially useful results of preoperative chemotherapy have been discussed. These are a consequence of effects on the primary tumor itself. Initial chemotherapy followed by delayed removal of the primary tumor allows the physician to assess the impact of the drug treatment on the tumor itself. Thus, one has an opportunity of directly studying the biology of chemotherapy-induced regression. Depending upon the magnitude of the response, this may allow the investigator to modify an initial drug treatment program so as to select more appropriate agents.

Finally, but not least important, a significant impact of chemotherapy on the primary tumor may permit the use of less extensive and destructive surgical procedures. Or, alternatively, it may allow the primary tumor to be more readily sterilized by follow-up radiation. Thus, initial chemotherapy may permit better local control with, at the same time, less radical procedures.

There would, therefore, appear to be many potential avenues of benefit for neoadjuvant chemotherapy, and it is certainly important that this modality be appropriately tested in properly designed clinical trials. There are a number of tantalizing hints from still incomplete studies as well as from uncontrolled clinical observations. It is vital, therefore, that definitive answers to questions of the utility of neoadjuvant treatment in a variety of human malignancies be evaluated.

Although there are logistic problems in pre- and perioperative chemotherapy, the possibility that control rates in certain cancers may be significantly enhanced makes this an attractive area for clinical investigation. The next few years should see some definitive answers emerging as to whether appropriate timing of adjuvant chemotherapy, even with existing drug protocols, can have a significant impact on cancer cure rates.

Subject Index

MIX
Papier aus verantwortungsvollen Quellen
Paper from responsible sources
FSC® C105338

If you have any concerns about our products,
you can contact us on
ProductSafety@springernature.com

In case Publisher is established outside the EU,
the EU authorized representative is:
Springer Nature Customer Service Center GmbH
Europaplatz 3, 69115 Heidelberg, Germany

Printed by Libri Plureos GmbH
in Hamburg, Germany